Holistic Medicine

Holistic Medicine

A Meeting of East and West

HENRY EDWARD ALTENBERG, M.D.

Japan Publications, Inc.

Note to the reader: Those with health problems are advised to seek the guidance of a qualified medical or psychological professional before implementing any of the approaches presented in this book. It is essential that any readers who have any reason to suspect serious illness in themselves or their family members seek appropriate medical, nutritional, or psychological advise promptly. Neither this nor any other health-related books should be used as a substitute for qualified care or treatment.

Published by Japan Publications, Inc., Tokyo

Distributors:
UNITED STATES: Kodansha America, Inc., through Oxford University Press, 198 Madison Avenue, New York, N.Y. 10016. CANADA: Fitzhenry & Whiteside Ltd., 195 Allstate Parkway, Markham, Ontario L3R 4T8. UNITED KINGDOM AND EUROPEAN CONTINENT: Premier Book Marketing Ltd., 1 Gower Street, London WC1E 6HA. AUSTRALIA AND NEW ZEALAND: Bookwise International, 54 Crittenden Road, Findon, South Australia 5023. ASIA AND JAPAN: Japan Publications Trading Co., Ltd., 1-2-1, Sarugaku-cho, Chiyoda-ku, Tokyo 101. Japan.

First edition   : July 1992
Second printing : August 1998

ISBN 0-87040-902-6

Printed in U. S. A.

To Jean, whose intuition matches her wisdom

There is nothing more admirable than when two
people who see eye to eye keep house as husband and wife,
confounding their enemies and delighting their friends,
as they themselves know best.

HOMER
The Odyssey, Book VI

Acknowledgments

Fifteen years ago I made a brief pilgrimage to my childhood community to see the house where I had lived from four to twenty, and also paid a brief visit to the public school that I had attended from kindergarten to sixth grade. None of the teachers or principal were still there, after forty years. I asked to speak briefly to the principal, and thanked him as official representative of the school department for my earliest education, where I learned to read and write. I again wish to thank Public School 114 for the excellent primary education I received in those days. I was fortunate to obtain an equally competent education in high school and college.

I acknowledge the excellent basic medical education I received from my professors and teachers at New York University School of Medicine. Since then there have been many other teachers throughout my various postgraduate training experiences. I particularly wish to acknowledge Karl Menninger, M. D. as a mentor in my initial psychiatric training. Dr. Karl referred to himself as a "cockleburr under the saddle," goading his students to explore and remain open to new ideas.

I acknowledge Michio Kushi for his lectures, books and inspiration to seek One Peaceful World, and to create health and the healing of the ill. I am grateful for the sharing of their journey by the many individuals who have attended healing conferences and have been an inspiration in so many ways. I am especially appreciative of all the teaching that many have given me who have attended the support group meetings that I have participated in, either as observer or as co-facilitator.

I owe a debt of gratitude to those practitioners who kindly reviewed my chapters relating to their varied fields of expertise: Timothy Kingsbury, D. O. for his comments and help with osteopathy, William Kragen, D. C. for his constructive criticism and additions on chiropractic; Devra Krassner, N. D. for her assistance with naturopathy; Kristy Fassler, N. D. for her contributions on homeopathy, and Ayn Rose, R. P. P. for Polarity Therapy. I appreciate the faith and support of John Harvey Gray, Reiki Master. I wish to thank Mr. Yoshiro Fujiwara of Japan Publications for his confidence and advice during the past two years.

Above all, I wish to acknowledge my wife, Jean, not only for the encouragement I received, similar to what is frequently experienced by many other authors, but beyond that, her practical and concrete assistance in reading each chapter as it was written and giving honest and objective feedback. I now know why so many authors speak so highly of their wives. Truly, without the support and encouragement I received, this book could not have been written.

HENRY EDWARD ALTENBERG
Kittery, Maine
January 3, 1992

Source Acknowledgments

Grateful acknowledgment is made to the following for use of material from the following sources:

Austin, Phyllis. "We must humanize medicine." Topsham, ME: Maine Times. Copyright 22 Feb 91 by The Maine Times. Used by permission of Phyllis Austin.

Baginski, Bodo, and Shalila Sharamon. *Reiki: Universal Life Energy*. Used by permission of LifeRhythm, P.O. Box 806, Mendocino, California: Copyright 1988 by LifeRhythm.

Boucher, Joseph. "Naturopathic Medicine: a Separate and Distinct Healing Profession." *Wholistic Dimensions in Healing*. Ed. Leslie J. Kaslof. New York: Copyright 1978 by Doubleday.

Crampton, Martha. "Psychological Energy Transformations: Developing Positive Polarization." *Transpersonal Psychology* 6.1 (1974) Copyright 1974 by Transpersonal Institute. Used by permission of the publisher.

Engel, George. "The Need for a New Medical Model: A Challenge for Biomedicine." *Science*. 196: 8 Apr 1977

——. "The Clinical Application of the Biopsychosocial Model." *American Journal of Psychiatry*. 127: 535 (1980). Copyright 1980 by American Journal of Psychiatry

Flach, Frederic. *Rickie*. New York: Fawcett Columbine, 1990. Copyright 1990 by Frederic Flach, M.D. Used by permission of Random House, publishers.

Haberly, Helen. *Hawayo Takata's Story*. Garrett Park, Maryland: Archedigm, 1990. Copyright 1990 by Helen J. Haberly.

Hammer, Leon. *Dragon Rises, Red Bird Flies*. New York: Station Hill Press, 1990. Copyright 1990 by Leon I. Hammer, M.D.

Lock, Margaret. *East Asian Medicine in Urban Japan*. Berkeley, CA: University of California Press, 1980. Copyright 1980 by the Regents of the University of California.

Lucas, Richard. *Nature's Medicines*. Copyright 1966 by Parker Publishing Co., Inc. West Nyack, NY.

Norris, Patricia and Garrett Porter. *Why Me?: Harnessing the Healing Power of the Human Spirit*. Walpole, NH: Stillpoint Publishing, 1985. Copyright 1985 by Garrett Porter and Patricia A. Norris, Ph.D. Used by permission of the publisher.

Pelletier, Kenneth. *Holistic Medicine: From Stress to Optimum Health*. New York: Delacorte and Delta, 1979. Copyright 1979 by Kenneth R. Pelletier.

Sandler, Stephen. *Osteopathy, the Illustrated Guide*. New York: Harmony Books, 1989. Copyright 1989 by The Hamlyn Publishing Group Limited.

Shah, Idries. From TALES OF THE DERVISHES by Idries Shah. Copyright © 1967 by Idries Shah. Used by permission of the publisher, Dutton, an imprint of New American Library, a division of Penguin Books USA Inc.

Spiegel, David. "A Psychosocial Intervention and Survival Time of Patients with Metastatic Breast Cancer." *Advances, The Journal of Mind-Body Health*. 7: 3 (Summer 1991). Copyright 1991 by John E. Fetzer Institute. By permission of the publisher.

"The Surgeon General's Report on Nutrition and Health: The Summary and Recommendations." New York: Warner Books, 1989.

Tribe, Bill. "Naturopathic Medicine." From the *Holistic Health Handbook.* by the Berkeley Holistic Health Center. Copyright © 1978 by Edward Bauman, Armand Brint, Lorin Piper, and Pamela Wright. Used by permission of the Stephen Greene Press, an imprint of Penguin Books USA, Inc.

Tsumura, Akira. *Kampo: How the Japanese Updated Traditional Medicine*. Tokyo & New York: Japan Publications, Inc., 1991. Copyright 1991 by Akira Tsumura.

Veith, Ilza. *Nei Ching: The Yellow Emperor's Classic of Internal Medicine*. Berkeley, CA: University of California Press. Copyright © 1947, 1975 by Ilza Veith.

Weil, Andrew. *Health and Healing*. Boston: Houghton Mifflin, 1986. Copyright 1983, 1988 by Andrew Weil.

——. *Natural Health, Natural Medicine*. Boston: Houghton Mifflin, 1990. Copyright© 1990 by Andrew Weil, M.D. Reprinted by permission of Houghton Mifflin Company. All rights reserved.

Wild, Richard. "Chiropractic." Reprinted from *Hands-On Healing.* 1989 by Rodale Press, Inc. Permission granted by Rodale Press, Inc. Emmaus, PA 18098.

Wilhelm, Richard. *The I Ching*. Princeton, NJ: Princeton University Press. Copyright © 1950 by Bollingen Foundation.

Foreword

During my term as President of the American Holistic Medical Association in the late 1980's, I, like those before me, struggled with creating an inclusive vision for our members of what holistic medicine really was. All the members of the American Holistic Medical Association have been trained as M.D.s or D.O.s in conventional medical schools that by and large teach medicine as though our bodies were divided into distinct and separate non-interacting systems. In conventional medicine the mind/body dichotomy is so great that the mind is taken care of by psychiatrists while the rest of the body is divided among an ever-growing number of specialists. We must remember that this high-tech fragmentation of our bodies is consistent with the Newtonian world-view of Western industrialized culture. As Richard Sandor writes:

> The society clever enough to perform sophisticated research on cancer is the society clever enough to invent sugar substitutes, children's sleepwear ingredients, food-coloring agents, and swimming pool test kits that may cause it.*

My physician colleagues join the AHMA from all kinds of different specialties, mostly because they realize that something is missing in the way conventional medicine is taught and practiced, something that all of us inherently know, but have forgotten in this fragmented world: Our bodies are not made up of organ systems presided over by an authoritarian brain that is separate from our hearts, emotions, and spirits. We are instead a complex physical manifestation of our thoughts, dietary choices, relationships, parents, communities, hopes, and dreams. Our bodies and our states of health are determined by the interplay of countless variables that cannot be easily reduced to the simplistic cause and effect approach of allopathic medicine. Along with the AHMA during the 1980's the science of psychoneuroimmunology—the study of how the mind,

---

*David Ehrenfeld, "The Arrogance of Humanism" cited in the article "The Attending Physician." Richard S. Sandor, in *The Sun*, issue 190, Sept. 1991, pg.4.

nervous system, endocrine system, and immune systems are all interrelated—was also growing, lending scientific credence to what our intuition was already telling us.

As part of its evolution the AHMA developed its core curriculum areas: knowledge felt to represent holistic medicine that was not covered in medical school. Nutrition, self-regulation, exercise, homeopathy, and chelation therapy, as well as some others, were included. Every year practitioners of modalities such as chiropractic and herbology would complain that their techniques were not represented in the core curriculum. Every year we found ourselves in a defensive position. How could we call ourselves "holistic" if we weren't including lectures on massage therapy, for example, at our annual meeting? There were so many modalities, so many advocates of different healing systems! We were in danger of losing sight of the forest, as each of the "trees" lobbied for recognition and inclusion.

Was holistic medicine simply a group of techniques and approaches different from conventional, allopathic medicine: approaches that relied upon herbs and vitamins vs. drugs and surgery? Or was it more than that? Bernie Siegel, M. D., my co-President at the time, was practicing general surgery as his main healing technique. His modalities were those of a surgeon: anesthesia, high technology equipment, and surgical blades to cut out organs. Was THIS holistic?

All of us knew so-called "holistic" practitioners who treated everything as though it were a nutritional deficiency, simply because nutrition was their specialty—and still others, trained in psychology, who treated every problem as if it were emotionally based. Clearly, the concept "holistic" was much-used and little understood. Most of my patients had the idea that anything involving vitamins was holistic, but anything that required surgery was not. Where was the truth?

The board members of the AHMA finally arrived at a conclusion that made sense to everyone: Holism is not simply modalities that offer alternatives to drugs or surgery. Our conclusion was much more expansive and freeing than that.

Holism is a way of being in the world—an approach to the patient that acknowledges that she or he is more than a collection of organs and tissues that work mechanically like a machine. Holism acknowledges that each of us is greater than the sum or our individual parts—each of us is a hologram in which each part also reflects the whole.

Within this framework we also acknowledged that there were countless healing tools that could be used in service to our vision of healing the whole person. We elected, however, to drop our designation of core curriculum areas. We realized that we were not in a position to adequately represent all the various useful techniques employed by holistic practitioners. We decided instead to promote holism as a philosophy which supports many different healing tools, including drugs and surgery when appropriate. We acknowledged also that those with training in disciplines other than conventional medicine had much to offer those of us who did. Many of us work in partnership with healers of all kinds—acupuncturists, polarity therapists, chiropractors, herbal healers, and nutritionists, to name a few.

There is no reason why we can't have everything—the best of conventional medicine, and the best of the healing practices that Dr. Altenberg has illuminated for us in this book. We need to remember also that conventional medicine is very new—it has been around less than one hundred years. Some of the modalities explored in this book have stood the test of centuries. I, like Dr. Altenberg, have personally experienced and recommended many of them.

Most are spiritually-based approaches that acknowledge the inherent healing power within each of us—a power that is sorely needed at this time in human and planetary history. A new vision for health-care is urgently needed. Holistic medicine, both philosophy *and* modalities, will be a part of that vision. In her highly acclaimed book on the future, *The Popcorn Report,* Faith Popcorn, a consultant to the Fortune 500 companies, tells us that in the next decade, "Medical knowledge and alternatives will cross cultures in a way we have never seen before… holistic medicine will move from the fringes to the mainstream of medicine." I offer the following example of what that vision looks like in my office.

Several years ago a medical student from the University of Vermont was spending the morning at Women to Women as part of her obstetrics and gynecology rotation at our medical center. She watched and listened while I examined and spoke with my patients. While performing a uterine biopsy, I placed my hands over the patient's lower abdomen and did a technique called therapeutic touch. This helps restore the patient's energy field after an invasive procedure and also helps decrease the discomfort and fear that are so often a part of medical testing. While the patient was still lying on the examination table, I asked her to breathe regularly and simply pay attention to any thoughts or images that came up. Women often experience old memories following the placing of an instrument in the uterus. Unresolved grief about an abortion, or even memories of incest can sometimes surface. Telling my patients about this gives them permission to acknowledge how hurts are often stored in the body.

Several other patients that morning were given natural options for their gynecologic problems, such as dietary changes, food supplements, and castor oil packs. Some were treated with standard drugs such as estrogen replacement therapy. In every case I spent some time talking with the patient about what was going on in her life.

In my office later that morning, the medical student turned to me and said, "I'm confused. Yesterday you did a hysterectomy in the hospital. Now today in your office you are suggesting herbs to some people, surgery to others, and doing therapeutic touch in your exam room after a procedure. What is going on here?"

The student was experiencing a rather common error in thinking. She had the idea that surgery, the hospital, and standard medications wouldn't be used by the same doctor who used so-called "holistic" modalities such as therapeutic touch. I assured her that holistic medicine is really a mind set—a way of thinking about healing. At the heart of medicine what is most important is the consciousness of the doctor and his/her relationship with the patient.

Once this relationship is established, the particular modalities that a holistic doctor uses are highly variable and certainly might include drugs and surgery. Most holistic doctors, operating under the ancient dictum, "first, do no harm," will be more likely to use non-toxic methods whenever possible. Our dualistic culture with its either/or thinking leads us to believe that holistic medicine is contrary to conventional medicine or vice versa. I often have the experience while standing at the scrub sink in surgery of having a colleague say, "What are you doing here? Is this another failure of macrobiotics that you're operating on?" I keep a sense of humor and gently point out that I like to have it all: brown rice and anesthesia when necessary.

Though more and more people are interested in natural, non-toxic remedies and approaches, we need not lose the elegance of modern technological medicine. We need both. In the coming decades we'll see medical centers where the best aspects of all of medicine, ancient and modern, are joined together in systems of health-care that honor us as whole people: body, mind, spirit, community, and planet. It's time.

CHRISTIANE NORTHRUP, M.D., F.A.C.O.G.

*Fellow, American College of Obstetricians
    and Gynecologists*
*Past President, American Holistic Medical
    Association*
*Asst. Clinical Professor of Obstetrics and
    Gynecology, Univ. of Vermont College
    of Medicine*
*Co-Founder, Women to Women Healthcare
    Center, Yarmouth, Maine*

Preface

Since I graduated from medical school, I have practiced medicine in six of the United States and one territory. Beginning with my interneship year in Rhode Island, a year as a medical resident in Ohio, I next spent three years in Kansas as a psychiatric resident and staff psychiatrist. My two years in Alaska were at a time when it was still a territory. I then practiced in Connecticut for thirty years, until moving to Maine. For the past eight years I have been practicing in New Hampshire and Maine. Each of these states has granted me a license to practice as a Doctor of Medicine. The requirements to qualify for these licenses included graduation from an accredited medical school and the completion of at least one or two years of additional training as an interne or resident. None of the training I received as a resident in several programs had any relationship to holistic medicine. There are no formal or official training programs at this time in holistic medicine. There is no recognition of holistic medicine as any form of conventional medicine.

I do not know who was the first physician to declare that they were a holistic physician. In 1978 the American Holistic Medical Association was established. The only requirement is to be a licensed M.D. or D.O. (Doctor of Osteopathy), and have enough interest to pay dues and declare one's interest. Most physicians who have so identified themselves have pursued additional studies in a wide range of health subjects, either by self-study or through attending various lectures and courses on nutrition, herbal medicine, homeopathy, Chinese or Oriental medicine, acupuncture, or other non-conventional subjects.

This is different from the usual approach to medical specialization. Most physicians who have come to declare their holistic orientation do not consider themselves as specialists in holistic medicine. Some have acquired more extensive knowledge in certain subjects. As a result, they may limit their practice to the use of certain specialized techniques, such as nutrition, or homeopathy, but these are not conventionally defined specialties.

Holistic health is a close ally of holistic medicine. It is broad in scope and involves many non-medical practitioners and laypersons. Simultaneously, it has become a field of study and practice that has several concrete and specific forms. Herbalism is a field that draws from centuries of knowledge and practice from Europe, Asia, and Native American cultures. More laypersons are engaged in herbalism, or herbal medicine, than professionals, with the exception that most naturopathic physicians also treat many patients with herbs.

The field of psychotherapy is not usually defined as having any particular holistic characteristics. Some psychotherapists, however, have strong convictions that the mind and body cannot be separated. In varying degrees counseling can be used as part of the treatment for the healing of physical ailments. This is an element of a holistic viewpoint. There are also psychotherapists who have a strong leaning toward spiritual elements in their theory and practice. Transpersonal counseling and several other forms of counseling contain metaphysical elements. These also can be viewed as containing a holistic orientation. Some metaphysical counselors, such as Louise Hay or Rosalyn Bruyere, are not usually defined as "professional" and yet contribute a great deal to the public at large, and also to individuals who seek help from them or their associates. The use of books, audio and video tapes by Louise Hay, Shakti Gawain, Patricia Sun and others contribute to a broader approach to health: physical, mental and spiritual.

In ancient Greece, before Hippocrates, the father of modern, Western scientific medicine established the Rational school of medicine, there was a school of medicine called the Empirical School. It eventually lost its place to Hippocratic medicine. It has gained a negative and old-fashioned reputation, especially in the past several centuries, and most of all in the past hundred years. Holistic medicine is neither purely empirical nor is it predominantly scientific. In many respects a holistic viewpoint is part of the ethic and theory of modern medicine, concerning itself with the whole person: mind, body and spirit. Unfortunately, the holistic viewpoint gets lost in today's world of medical practice, which reflects many aspects of the modern culture in which it is practiced. Modern scientific medicine in its application is increasingly rushing, under pressure, with an increasing alienation between practitioner and patient. The patient continues to become more impatient, and the physician suffers too often from irritability, frustration, and anxiousness.

Holistic thinking about health and illness proposes more self-responsibility and greater partnership between patient and doctor. It also seeks a greater interest in maintaining a health that is not only the absence of disease, but seeks to strive for a level of wellness that ideally is "high-level wellness," as proposed by Don Ardell (Ardell, 1977) and John Travis, M.D. Holistic medicine attempts to be open-minded toward healing practices of other cultures, though not scientifically yet proven. It has a degree of comfort with empirical methods. Holistic medicine does not exclude an awareness of Spirit or Soul, and the religious dimension. Meaning and purpose in all aspects of life have a connection to healing. This includes the search for meaning and purpose in illness and disease, death and dying. Holistic medicine is, at its best, like conventional medicine, a caring medicine, that participates equally in the relief of suffering and impairment.

The purpose of this book is to be a guidebook—akin to a travel guidebook—to allow the general reader to become more aware of how much exists in the world at large, at home and in other countries. A major goal is to help individuals to maintain health, and to enhance healing, with or without conventional medical care. This is more of a sampler than a complete guidebook. The field of holistic health and medicine includes other methods that are not included here.

Anyone with a health problem should not try to use any comments in this book as a form of diagnosis or treatment, but should consult an appropriate health professional. I do not propose that anyone should avoid or shun conventional medical care. Some life-threatening conditions demand immediate attention, for which only a competent medical doctor can properly help.

More than twenty years ago I received a reply to a letter I had sent to the editor of the *Archives of Psychiatry and Neurology*. It was in response to my questioning the bias of a book reviewer, who had severely criticized the author of a book on group psychotherapy. The author was a highly popular and successful psychiatrist-writer. He had written in a clear and non-technical manner about a serious subject. The editor's rebuttal to me stated, "Anyone who writes for the public is not writing for the scientist." I hope that I have fulfilled a proper obligation in writing for the public. If health professionals or others committed to the scientific method find some useful information here, I shall be happy to have included both groups as readers. If not, then I shall be content if the general reader finds satisfaction in what follows.

HENRY EDWARD ALTENBERG, M.D.

Then came a man of knowledge, who said to the merchants of tea, and the drinkers of tea, and to others: "He who tastes, knows. He who tastes not, knows not. Instead of talking about the celestial beverage, say nothing, but offer it at your banquets. Those who like it will ask for more. Those who do not, will show that they are not fitted to be tea-drinkers. Close the shop of argument and mystery. Open the teahouse of experience." And those who tasted, knew.

—from the teachings of the Master Hamadani, died 1140.

Contents

PART III

Non-Medical Healing: Eastern and Western

PART IV

Twenty-First Century Medicine

I

Western Traditions of Healing

1
Personal Journey

I was born in New York City and lived there for the first sixteen years of my life. I was fortunate to have some contact with non-urban Nature. For some years we lived on the south shore of Long Island, a few hundred yards from the Atlantic Ocean. I could hear the surf breaking on the shore from my bedroom window.

I also went to an overnight camp in Maine every summer from the age of seven to ten. This experience had a strong imprint on me in several ways. I recall my first exposure to the visual beauty of a Maine lake surrounded by pine trees and the smell of pine needles. It was a well-run camp with friendly counselors, each of whom we called Uncle Steve or Uncle Bill, or whatever their first names were. Besides the counselors there was a Penobscot Indian from Old Town, Maine who was on the staff to teach and speak about Indian lore. The memory of my contacts with Chief Lone Wolf has remained fresh in my mind. I have no idea if he was an authentic tribal chief, but he was a member of the Penobscot tribe.

My memory of his face has dimmed, but I clearly recall frequently spending time sitting with him in the woods, with few words exchanged. He was not only a real person to me but he also had some qualities of The Wise Old Man archetype, as described by Carl Jung. I have always felt that I had experienced some special connection. Yet, I wondered. I have thought about that experience at the age of seven from time to time.

Almost sixty years later, in 1991, an unusual event occurred, unlike any I have ever heard described. One camper, now a businessman in his fifties or possibly older, decided to organize a reunion of campers who had attended this camp. It had not been in operation for the past fifty years. He was successful in contacting many ex-campers despite the years that had passed. Forty-eight campers and their wives and friends attended, including myself.

Several annual yearbooks that the camp published were available to browse through at the reunion. I saw and read three of the yearbooks for the years I had attended. In the one for the year when I was seven there was a description of each camper and his cabin mates. The counselor's description of me mentioned my close contact with Chief Lone Wolf. I could confirm my memory of half a century ago! Chief Lone Wolf also was in a photograph.

This contact with Lone Wolf had imprinted enough on me, I believe, to encourage explorations later into studying different cultures, i.e., cultural anthropology, that has persisted to this day. It has been a source of curiosity for me that has also led to the subject of this book. I began to read about Native Americans in my early adolescence. While living in New York City then, I could often visit several museums. I was within walking distance of the Museum of Natural History. The rooms full of totem poles and other Native American objects fascinated me. I fantasized becoming an anthropologist.

On one occasion I asked to meet with a staff anthropologist at the museum to ask how I might become an anthropologist. She agreed to meet me and was accepting of a fifteen-year old boy asking for information. Her not too surprising advice was to go to college and then study in graduate school. I thanked Margaret Mead and went back to look at the exhibits.

In that same year I went on a bicycle trip that traveled through the Southwest United States. I saw Pueblo Indians for the first time in Santa Fé, New Mexico. The following year I returned to New Mexico and attended the University of New Mexico Field School of Anthropology and Archeology.

About seven of the students, including myself, visited Navaho homes on the Navaho Indian reservation at Chaco Canyon, New Mexico as part of the study of anthropological field techniques. The rest of the students participated in archeological excavation of eleventh century Pueblo ruins. Although this program of field work was primarily for graduate students, I participated as a non-credit student. I learned about and observed some traditional Navaho healing ceremonies, a blend of healing and religious ceremony conducted by a tribal medicine man. I didn't know it at the time, but I was observing an example of holistic medicine and healing for the first time. While still in medical school I managed to return to the Navaho reservation for another summer. This time I worked as an externe, or medical student assistant, in a Presbyterian mission hospital in Ganado, Arizona. Most of the patients were Navaho and Hopi, and a few were "Anglos" from local trading posts or from the mission compound.

My interest in anthropology has continued since then. I could not study it in my undergraduate college years, since the college did not offer courses in anthropology and I had become a pre-medical student. That required a focus on biology and chemistry with little time for social sciences, especially with an accelerated program during World War II. That program moved pre-medical students into medical school after only three years of college.

During my third year of medical school I enrolled at Columbia University in a course titled "Personal counseling for religious workers." This was entirely separate from my regular medical studies at New York University School of Medicine. The instructor for the course was Otis Rice, Episcopal chaplain at St. Luke's Hospital, near Columbia University. Most of the class were women preparing to be social workers in the Episcopal Church. The rest of us had a more general interest in counseling.

Otis Rice was an excellent lecturer, highly knowledgeable and enthusiastic about psychology. He taught the class some of Carl Jung's ideas. Besides the formal lectures we had an opportunity to get some practical experience by going onto the medical and surgical wards of St. Luke's Hospital at least one afternoon a week as a chaplain's assistant.

Despite my schedule at the medical school I managed to "sneak off" to St. Luke's Hospital. I presented myself as a chaplain's assistant, wearing a half-length white coat with a small purple cross on it. I would then speak to several patients on the wards. Despite my youthfulness I managed to look serious and studious enough to engage the patients. The patients felt distressed enough to share with me some of their complaints and dislikes. Their chief subject was the way some of the doctors and nurses dealt with them. I also talked with the nurses who told me about some of their struggles with the more "difficult" patients.

I gained some viewpoints that I didn't learn in my medical school classes or on the wards of Bellevue Hospital. As part of my training I went on the wards in a long white coat as a medical student to examine patients with a stethoscope and tongue depressors. The chaplain's role had given me a viewpoint about medicine I could not get as a medical student. There the focus was mostly on deciding if the patient in bed number six had an enlarged liver. There were a few courses in psychiatry but limited in scope. The emphasis was on severe mental illness. Psychological factors in physical illness were not given much attention at all.

After medical school the next step was to go through an interneship. This was to be for at least a year before entering any specialty training or entering general practice. I did this and then spent a year as a resident in internal medicine before starting a three-year residency in psychiatry.

During the year as a medical resident in Ohio, I participated in the treatment of patients with various medical conditions, such as heart disease, kidney disease, and lung disease. My interest in psychiatry also grew. I gave simple pencil and paper psychological tests to several patients. I became increasingly aware of the role of personality factors in physical illness.

My interest in anthropology continued, especially cultural anthropology. One contribution of anthropology was to alert me to systems, such as family systems, organizational systems, and the interrelationship of different parts of a culture. This helped me to remain open to non-scientific ways of thinking, in contrast to medical education and biological science training.

Psychiatry for me was a form of applied anthropology. For all my three years as a psychiatric resident the split between mind and body was strong. I abandoned the stethoscope I had used for the previous six years as a medical student, interne, and medical resident. My tools became my eyes, ears, and speech. Although there was some communication with physicians outside the field of psychiatry, there was a sense that I was in a different world. Now I was dealing with the mind and emotions, but little to no direct dealings with the body.

The term, psychosomatic medicine, had become popular for awhile while I was in medical school and for a decade later. It still exists, but the earlier enthusiasm has disappeared. Some researchers correlated certain personality features with specific diseases, such as high blood pressure, stomach ulcers, and arthritis. Since exact statistics could not prove the correlation, the ideas and interest decreased for a long time. Only in recent years with new research has there been a return to an interest in the relationship of emotions and physical illness.

I remember hearing Hans Selye, M.D. in 1947 lecture on his new ideas on the effects of stress on the physical condition of laboratory animals. I speculated that his research would become of importance in the next forty years. Selye eventually acquired the title of "the Father of Stress." I heard him lecture again thirty years later, in his seventies. The everyday practice of medicine in 1977 had still not fully accepted nor applied his ideas. Research and scientific articles in the past ten to fifteen years, however, have underlined the importance of his work. The new field of psychoneuroimmunology particularly supports Selye's findings.

Shortly after completion of psychiatric residency the United States Air Force assigned me as psychiatrist for the northern half of Alaska, based in Fairbanks, Alaska. I next settled in Connecticut, began a practice in psychotherapy and office-based psychiatry, also consultation work with a few social agencies. An interest in child psychiatry led to a part-time position in a child guidance clinic. A few years later I returned for a seventeen-month residency in child psychiatry in Worcester, Massachusetts.

Throughout the thirty years of practice in Connecticut, I was never totally satisfied with the theories and methods I had learned from training, study, and reading. I kept looking. I attended a variety of conferences and workshops to hear what was happening at the frontiers. One organization that was constantly presenting and sharing new directions in psychotherapy was the American Academy of Psychotherapists. Their summer workshops and annual conferences were innovative and thought-provoking for several decades.

Two annual conferences, in 1967 and 1972, presented speakers who significantly stimulated holistic thinking. The 1967 conference, *Comparative Systems of Healing,* was not only about psychotherapy but dealt with healing systems in a variety of ways. Both Eastern and Western healing systems had spokespersons. An East Indian Kali healer from Guyana, South America, shared his work, followed by a discussion by an anthropologist. A chiropractor, a Christian Scientist and a conventional psychotherapist also gave summaries of their work, with a discussant for each of their presentations.

The following day each speaker met with a small group of attenders who chose to hear them. I attended the session of the chiropractor. He was the first chiropractor I had ever seen or heard. I lacked previous information or teaching about chiropractic that might have led me to understand it better. I was familiar with the American Medical Association's declaration for years that defined chiropractic as "unproven, unscientific" and therefore considered as "quackery."

I shall leave the details of my happy encounter with the chiropractor at this conference for a later chapter. It was a highly enlightening and unstiffening experience. In recent years the A.M.A. has changed its viewpoint officially and does not discourage or forbid conventional physicians from referring to chiropractors.

In 1972 the Academy of Psychotherapists held their annual conference on "Beyond the Senses." This was a mind-boggling experience. The meeting included presenters on parapsychology, astrology, Yoga, and the sentience or "feelings" of plants. I also heard Lawrence LeShan, Ph.D. speak on the similarities in ideas between mystics and small-particle physicists. He also spoke about studies of nonconventional healers, such as spiritual healers who did hands-on healing, or "laying on of hands." This was before Dolores Krieger had written her book, *Therapeutic Touch* (Krieger, 1979).

Several years later I heard about Dr. LeShan's extensive psychotherapeutic work with cancer patients over a thirty-five year period. He has described this in *Cancer as a Turning Point* (LeShan, 1989).

In the early 1970s several organizations began to explore broader realms of healing than found within conventional medicine. The Academy of Parapsychology and Medicine, based in California, published the talks given at the 1971 and 1972 annual meetings. I could then read the first presentation by Carl Simonton, M. D., a radiation oncologist. He included visualization techniques as a supplement to radiation therapy for people with advanced or terminal cancers. He has continued this work over the following twenty years.

Other presentations included Elmer Green, Ph. D., a major researcher on biofeedback and the voluntary control of involuntary states. Published reports appeared of more unusual forms of nonconventional healing. Holistic health and medicine were clearly gestating into their births. Another organization, The Association for Holistic Health in California, published talks given at its meetings in 1975 and 1976.

The Wellness movement also appeared on the scene in California in the 1970s. I attended a workshop in 1978 given by John Travis, M. D., who had started the first private practice for wellness in Mill Valley, California. The workshop he gave in Baltimore, Maryland in 1978 was on Stress Reduction and Burnout Prevention for health workers. This was the same year that Norman Shealy, M. D. founded the American Holistic Medical Association. Dr. Shealy is a neurosurgeon, presently the director of the Shealy Institute for Comprehensive Pain and Health Care in Springfield, Missouri, and president of Holos Institute of Health.

The Travis workshop was not only about the prevention of burnout, or exhaustion at work, but equally applicable to all aspects of life. My timing in attending this was fortunate, since I was soon to face the fact of my first wife's diagnosis of pancreatic cancer. That occurred two months later.

Her first symptoms had started gradually and with no hint of what would eventually occur. After consulting five different physicians and after many tests, a diagnosis was established in December of 1978. It was an inoperable condition. It had its usual rapid rush to a terminal state. In the fourteen years since then, the diagnosis and treatment of pancreatic cancer still is difficult and treatment minimally effective.

In the short period of four months from diagnosis to death, I came to learn about some nonconventional, alternative or complementary therapies for cancer. Although some of these complementary methods were used (but not as a substitute for conventional therapy), there was no response from either conventional or complementary methods. Nonetheless, I found the exploration a source of hope. I also learned that the field of nonconventional therapies is a large one, even a confusing one at times. My explorations had scarcely begun.

Many nonconventional approaches have reports of apparent cures, sometimes called by conventional physicians "spontaneous remissions." Most of these are still today considered unproven by standard scientific criteria, and usually physicians do not recommend them. Future research and more detailed reports may eventually sort out what can be useful and what is apparently useless.

An organization that also presented news from the frontiers has been the American Association for Humanistic Psychology. I first attended one of their annual meetings in 1968 in San Francisco. I attended several annual meetings after that, and made another discovery. At the 1970 annual meeting in Miami, Florida, Malcolm Brown, Ph. D. presented a demonstration of "Direct Body-contact psychotherapy" (Brown, 1990).

The title was intriguing for someone who had been heavily trained in "head" work and intellectual pursuits ever since grade school and for the next thirty years. Malcolm Brown spoke and demonstrated a psychotherapeutic approach that included working with and on the body. He had integrated methods and principles derived partly from Wilhelm Reich, M. D., Alexander Lowen, M. D. and also influenced by Carl Rogers, Carl Jung and D. H. Lawrence. Dr. Lowen had derived his system, known as Bioenergetic Analysis, from his study with Reich. Malcolm Brown has described his approach in *The Healing Touch* (Brown, 1990).

Watching Malcolm Brown present his methods inspired me. I felt somewhat like St.Paul on the road to Damascus. It was not exactly a conversion but definitely a profound challenge. I experienced a strong urge to pursue this direction. Shortly after the meeting I contacted a psychiatrist I had known a few years earlier. I knew he had some connection with Dr. Alexander Lowen in New York City.

Because of this renewed contact, I received an invitation to hear and observe Dr. Lowen at several seminars in New York City. In 1971 I entered a five-year training program in Bioenergetic Analysis with Dr. Lowen as both a teacher and my bioenergetic therapist. Both Reich, Lowen, and Malcolm Brown have demonstrated the unity of mind and body. Although none of them speak of holism in their writings, nonetheless, they are contributors to a more holistic approach for mind and body healing.

Alexander Lowen has described his work with several cancer patients who had been given a limited life span, but achieved complete remission of their cancers, after including bioenergetic therapy as part of their healing program (Lowen, 1987). Most of Lowen's bioenergetic therapy has dealt with treating psychological problems more than physical illness. Wilhem Reich years before in 1942 had written about cancer (Reich, 1973), and was decades ahead of his time in proposing a psychological view of cancer, both as causation and for treatment. He related some cancers to the psychological state of deep resignation.

Besides my professional concerns, the continuing interest in anthropology had given me some appreciation of religious ceremonies and practices throughout the world. I wanted to know how different cultures approached the spiritual aspects of life. I had also been searching for answers about Spirit since a young age. That was an element in my seeking Chief Lone Wolf when I was seven.

When I found writings that appeared to combine some aspects of Western psychology with religious or spiritual teachings, I wanted to read more. In the early 1960s I discovered Alan Watts. He was an excellent writer on Zen Buddhism and had been for several decades, continuing until his death in 1973. *Psychotherapy East and West* (Watts, 1961) was particularly intriguing, and conveyed the overlap of psychology and Zen Buddhism. Five months before he died, I had the opportunity to spend a weekend with him when he led a workshop on Zen meditation. He also gave an introduction to Taoism, which had also appealed to him, as it did for many others.

Since then I have read and experienced some aspects of Tibetan Buddhism, Sufism, and Yoga through seminars, retreats, and workshops. Following the "psychedelic" era of the 1960s, many Americans began to study Eastern teachings, and continue to do so. Richard Alpert, Ph. D., also known as Ram Das, has lectured extensively for the past twenty-five years throughout the United States. He has many perceptions and experiences of Eastern spiritual traditions, especially the Hindu tradition.

Ram Das first gained notoriety as a professor of psychology. Harvard University expelled him and Timothy Leary, because of their participation in the use of LSD. Dr. Alpert later traveled to India where he became a disciple of Neem Karoli Baba, a north Indian teacher and guru. After several years Alpert, as Ram Das, began lecturing throughout the United States.

I have listened to many of his audiotapes over the past twenty years, and have attended several of his workshops. He has also written several highly readable books. His ability to integrate Western psychology and spiritual teachings is outstanding, and useful. His distinctly well-preserved sense of humor and humility combined with high intelligence and sincerity make him a resource for holistic thinking. He has been lecturing for more than twenty years. Some of his earlier talks have been printed as *Be Here Now* (Ram Das, 1971) and *The Only Dance There Is* (Ram Das, 1974).

After my first wife's death from cancer, I became interested in a newly developing phenomenon, support groups for patients and families who were coping with life-threatening illnesses. I also developed a professional interest in the subject of death and dying, after facing these issues on a personal level. I met Dr. Elizabeth Kubler-Ross and started to read her contributions. These had never been a part of psychiatry before her explorations, leading to her first book, *On Death and Dying* (Kubler-Ross,1969). She had developed a five-day workshop called *Life, Death and Transition,* that she and some of her associates presented in different areas of the United States, Europe, and Australia. I participated in one given by her in Alfred, Maine in 1985.

A few years earlier I heard presentations about the support groups developed at the Center for Attitudinal Healing in Tiburon, California by Gerald Jampolsky, M.D., a child psychiatrist. This center has become a model for dozens of similar centers throughout the United States, Canada and several European countries. Dr. Jampolsky has written several books growing out of his spiritual journey, of which the Center was one expression. I have visited the Center several times and tried to start a similar center while still living in Connecticut.

Another support group organization that I learned about and observed while in Connecticut was Make Today Count. This group was started in the 1970s by Orville Kelley, an "atomic" army veteran who developed a lymphoma. It is now a national organization that helps people start groups to give emotional support to anyone with life-threatening illnesses of any kind. Bernard Siegel, M. D., a New Haven, Connecticut surgeon, has become nationally and internationally known for his books and support group organization, ECaP, Exceptional Cancer Patients. I shall speak of these in more detail in a later chapter.

In 1986 my professional and intellectual interests in holistic medicine shifted gears suddenly. I received a diagnosis of a thyroid tumor in the left lobe of my thyroid gland. I had not had any symptoms suggesting this at all. I had consulted my family practitioner because of some mild but persistent neck pain on the right side due to a flare-up of neck arthritis. This hadn't bothered me for thirty-three years, since the time I had been in the Air Force, at the age of twenty-seven.

Because the pain had persisted for about two weeks I decided to "run it by" the family doctor. I had learned years before there was nothing to do for it other than an occasional aspirin if it bothered me. Being older now I thought I would have it reevaluated. I learned that the acute episode is usually self-limiting. It quiets down with time and more aspirin, or the more recent successors to aspirin, such as Advil, Motrin, or Tylenol.

The doctor did suggest rechecking my neck with x-rays, which he then ordered. As I was about to leave the office, he placed his hands on my throat and asked me to swallow.

"Hmm," he said. "It almost feels like a slight hint of a swelling on the left side. We can wait a few weeks, but—since you're getting some x-rays anyway—let's have you get a radioactive scan of your thyroid gland."

There was no apparent connection between the questionable swelling on the left and the mild pain on the right. A week later the radioactive scan showed an egg-sized tumor in the left lobe of the thyroid. I saw a surgeon a short time later. Within another two weeks I underwent a partial thyroidectomy, which left the right lobe intact. The tumor would have eventually grown to the point that the swelling would have been obvious. It also might have caused difficulty in swallowing, if it pressed inward instead of outward.

The report from the pathologist after surgery revealed that it was a benign tumor, or adenoma. It was not quite as harmless as that term usually implies, since it had started to show a change toward becoming an adenocarcinoma, or cancer. It would have become so if its discovery had not occurred at that time. I have described this experience in more detail in *Doctors Look at Macrobiotics,* in a chapter entitled, "My Explorations in Macrobiotics."

Surgery was considered a cure. Nonetheless, I received the recommendation that I take a small amount of thyroid hormone for the rest of my life, to discourage the possibility of another tumor developing in the remaining lobe. There was no lack of thyroid hormone produced by the remaining lobe. Taking external hormone would cause the remaining lobe to hibernate like a bear in winter, and "lay low."

Once the doctor established a diagnosis, I suddenly recalled an event that had clear significance for the present situation. I had never mentioned it in any medical examinations in the past when I gave a medical history, since it hardly seemed worth mentioning. When I was about thirteen or fourteen, my adolescent acne was obvious. It was a mild case by most standards. I have no recollection that it was any worse than what had been true for my two older brothers. Nonetheless, my father sent me to a dermatologist who gave me at least two or possibly three x-ray treatments to my face.

I do not recall that the dermatologist used a neck shield in those days. The thyroid gland is one of the most sensitive parts of the body to radiation exposure. The Chernobyl explosion in the Soviet Union clearly proved this. Strontium-90, a substance released into the atmosphere by the Chernobyl explosion, was detected thousands of miles away, and is a major risk factor in causing future thyroid tumors.

Because of my thyroid tumor, I became much more personally interested in maintaining good health, and learning more about how to enhance it. I happened to discover several books on macrobiotics in a health food store shortly before my surgery. *Recalled by Life,* by Anthony Sattilaro, M.D. was particularly impressive, since the author was a physician who had been barely coping with metastatic prostate cancer (Sattilaro, 1982). I also purchased a macrobiotic cookbook. I later attended four of the annual summer conferences sponsored by the Kushi Foundation of Brookline, Massachusetts from 1986 to 1989.

In 1987 the editor of *Doctors Look at Macrobiotics* asked me to contribute an essay about my views on macrobiotics to be included in the book, later published in 1988 (Altenberg, 1988). In the following year the publishers asked me to write a book on holistic medicine, this present volume.

In 1988 my wife, Jean, and I created the Spruce Creek Holistic Center. We have sponsored lectures and workshops on a variety of health and healing topics by health professionals and other holistically oriented persons. We have also given workshops, and presently conduct a support group for anyone with life-threatening or serious physical illnesses.

During these four years we have met several hundreds of citizens. They have shared their thoughts and experiences, being not only clients and enrollees in workshops, but also teachers to us. We have also counseled some people to seek other methods for health enhancement and healing, besides their conventional medical treatments. We have never advised anyone to stop their conventional therapies. Some had already chosen to do so before we met them, or as they explored alternatives. This was especially true when conventional medicine lacked any specific treatment to offer, or the person had already received whatever conventional medicine and surgery could make available.

The journey continues. New books are constantly being published besides this one. The frontiers are constantly being pushed out in many directions throughout the world. My wife has a button she sometimes wears that states: "The possibilities are endless."

2

Holistic Medicine and Conventional Medicine

In the United States and in most of the industrialized countries of the world, the term, medical care, usually means the diagnosis and treatment of diseases by physicians, or Doctors of Medicine (M. D.), who are trained in a scientifically based system of study. Some writers call this traditional or conventional medicine. I prefer "conventional," since "traditional" in some parts of the world refers to what has been in use for many centuries, and is not usually based on a modern scientific viewpoint. A less common term for conventional, technologically based or Western medicine, is "allopathic" in contrast to "homeopathic." I shall discuss the origins of these terms later in my discussion of homeopathy.

Western medicine is also a common term for modern, scientifically-based medicine, in contrast to Eastern medicine. The difficulty with this term is that present-day India, Japan, and China use modern medical practice as much as in the geographical West. There are also systems of medical care used by citizens in the West that are not part of conventional medicine. Therefore, throughout this book I shall refer to the mainstream type of medical care as conventional, regardless of where the practice occurs. From this viewpoint other systems are likely to be viewed as nonconventional, except by those who always use them. As in politics or other human endeavors, your perspective may define what is normal or reasonable.

For the average American it is not easy to imagine that other systems of medical care exist besides the familiar conventional one. A few people are treated exclusively by Osteopathic physicians, who have a D. O. degree. A smaller number of people consult Naturopathic physicians, whose degree is N. D. Compared to the four hundred thousand M. D.s in the United States, there only thirty thousand chiropractic physicians, with a D. C. degree. Still less common are Doctors of Oriental Medicine (O. M. D.). Most of these are Chinese, but a few Americans have obtained this degree either in China or in schools of Oriental Medicine in the United States.

Osteopathic physicians may do surgery and prescribe pharmaceutical drugs. The others do not do surgery nor prescribe drugs. They may dispense or recommend herbal remedies, or specific nutritional substances, and use other methods such as physical manipulation of the body or the insertion of acupuncture needles. Despite the small number of M. D.s trained in acupuncture, some state laws only permit M. D.s to do acupuncture. In many states a licensed nonmedical acupuncturist may administer such treatments.

Having referred to several nonconventional healing systems, I wish to include a system of medical care that exists in India, where it had its origins, but is also practiced in the United States. This is Ayurveda, or Ayurvedic medicine. There is now an American Association of Ayurvedic Medicine with several hundred Western physicians who have received additional training in Ayurvedic medicine.

There are also many procedures and practices that are useful for health enhancement and for the healing of illnesses that nonmedical practitioners carry out. Examples are Rolfing, herbal remedies, massage therapy, and a variety of nutritional programs such as macrobiotics and wheat grass therapy. Some of these are supplements to conventional health care, while others are employed independently and may be controversial. Due to lack of scientific confirmation of their value some have been called not only unproven but dangerous, or viewed by some critics as quackery. The list of practices within the spectrum of holistic health is extensive.

Where does holistic medicine fit into conventional or nonconventional medicine? What is holistic medicine? Is it safe? These are important questions that require an answer. There is no single definition of holistic medicine that can satisfy everyone. There is no specialty by this name nor is it recognized officially as a specific set of principles or practices. The American Holistic Medical Association has existed since 1978 with a small number of M. D.s and D. O.s. There are now similar organizations in Japan, England, and Canada. There is also an American Holistic Nurses Association and a Canadian Holistic Nurses Association. In 1985 in England a Council for Complementary and Alternative Medicine came into being, with 1,250 members.

The word, holistic, is derived from "holism," a term coined in 1926 by the South African biologist-stateman, Jan Smuts. He was also the first prime minister of South Africa. In his book, *Holism and Evolution,* he proposed a new concept about living systems, suggesting that parts of a system are constantly moving toward larger wholes, greater than the sum of the parts that make it up. Holistic, in recent years, has also been spelled "wholistic," to emphasize its connection to wholeness.

Wholeness is a term that has been used in both a religious or spiritual context and in the psychology of Self, as in the writings of Roberto Assagioli, M.D. and Abraham Maslow. There is a connection between health and wholeness that is not apparent in the words themselves. Interestingly the origin of the English words gives a clue. The original old Anglo-Saxon word, *haelen,* which eventually became "health" and "heal," also contributed to the words "hale, hearty, holy" and "whole." The New Testament, originally written in Greek, contains the story of a woman with a menstrual illness who touches the hem of Jesus' robe (Luke 8:48) and is healed.

In the King James translation into English she is told: "Thy faith hath made thee whole." In several modern versions of the same passage, the passage reads: " Thy faith has made you well."

This suggests that wellness is wholeness. What then is wholeness? As it is commonly defined in holistic medicine, for example in the definition given by the American Holistic Medical Association, it is more than just physical wellness.

> Holistic medicine is a system of medical care that emphasizes personal responsibility and fosters a cooperative relationship among all those involved. It encompasses all safe modalities of diagnosis and treatment while emphasizing the whole person—physical, emotional and spiritual. Environmental, nutritional and life-style factors are also considered.

Holistic medicine is a coat of many colors. It is a term that is barely thirty years old, when applied to health and healing. It came into use in the late 1960s in California and early 1970s, and applied to health as well as illness or medical treatment. Both supporters and detractors alike perceived it sometimes as antagonistic to conventional medicine. Much if not all scientific medical research and medical practice is based on analytic studies of smaller and smaller particles, such as cells, nuclei of cells, and even smaller elements, such as genes. Holistic thinking emphasizes the larger and larger sweep of the body, mind, emotions and spirit. This moves it into the realm of less measurable elements and wholes, out of the realm of science and technology.

The strongest criticism of anything associated with holistic medicine is its unscientific position. This is true in several respects. The question for both practitioners and citizens, therefore, is how comfortable and acceptable is the use of ideas and methods that have not been proven or acceptable to science? The actual practice of medicine is both an art and a science. Conventional medical practitioners will only use methods that have been documented by scientific study. One decade's science, however, may turn out to be the next decade's disaster, because of new information. This is not to dismiss science, but merely to point out that errors do occur in science and research. The thalidomide disaster is one example, and the use of diethylstilbestrol, an estrogen hormone, is another. In the case of DES, daughters born to women who had been given estrogen to prevent early miscarriage had a high incidence later of vaginal cancer, related to the use of DES. My own experience of having x-ray radiation for adolescent acne is another example of acceptable medical practice eventually being incorrect and dangerous. This still leaves a major truth about holistic medicine that some of its practices are not acceptable to conventional medicine because of the lack of proofs.

Alternative medicine and complementary medicine are two terms that are used to refer to some of holistic medical practices. The British Council uses both terms. Complementary medicine suggests that holistic practices can be incorporated into the orthodox or mainstream practice of medicine. It also includes the acceptance of nonconventional methods by nonmedical health practitioners. Alternative medicine implies the use of methods that are in place of conventional medical care.

A more cautious view of holistic medicine sees it as adding a stronger emphasis on health promotion and patient education to conventional medical practice. A greater sense of partnership with the practitioner, and also more self-responsibility, without blame, is urged.

There have been several forces contributing to the increasing interest by the public in holistic medicine over the past twenty-five years. James Gordon, M. D. points out some of these in *Holistic Medicine* (Gordon, 1988) as he describes briefly the consumer rights movement, the ecology movement, and advances in psychology and psychiatry. Simultaneously there are the many crises in medical care financing, availability, and the problems of a breakdown in doctor-patient relationships. These in turn are moving citizens to search for answers beyond conventional and familiar medical care. This is not yet a large trend, but will increase over the coming decades.

The founder of the American Holistic Medical Association, Norman Shealy, M. D., trained and practiced for some years as a neurosurgeon. I have heard him speak of the change in his career from a busy neurosurgeon who operated on many patients with severe back problems to a physician who gave up performing surgery. He then developed and applied fewer invasive techniques for relieving pain. These included the use of stress reduction techniques, exercise, nutrition, and meditation, common forms of holistic practices. Obviously, they can be given or prescribed by conventional physicians, not only by those who define themselves as holistic. Many holistic approaches are not necessarily revolutionary or radical at all, at times part of medical practice but were swept away in the increasing technological tide of modern medicine.

Hippocrates, the ancient Greek physician, has the reputation of being the "Father of medicine." Scholars consider his writings more those of a group of physicians instead of one person, but the principles are still worthy of attention. Hippocrates stated "It is more important to know the person who has the disease than the disease the person has." Sir William Osler frequently quoted this statement. Dr. Osler was an outstanding professor of medicine in the early twentieth century. In the face of all the advances in technology it might be tempting for many medical practitioners to dismiss this as no longer useful. The exact opposite is true, as the close connections between emotions, mind, and bodily processes are becoming better understood. Sir William Osler knew that the tubercle bacillus was the bacteria that was necessary for the development of tuberculosis. Nonetheless he also said that the patient with tuberculosis needed to "have the head studied as much as the chest."

Kenneth Pelletier, Ph. D. in *Holistic Medicine* (Pelletier,1980) is firm in his conviction that "All states of health and all disorders are considered to be psychosomatic." He also writes: "Fundamental to holistic medicine is the recognition that each state of health and disease requires a consideration of all contributing factors: psychological, psychosocial, environmental, and spiritual." This is an alternative view of medicine, which has yet to be fully incorporated into the actual practice of medicine by most practitioners. Some conservative philosophers of science have declared this view "a patent falsehood." I don't agree.

The English poet, W. H. Auden, coined the phrase, The Age of Anxiety, to refer to much of the twentieth century after World War II. This expresses as much truth as poetry. Poets and other imaginative writers often express intuitively what scientists may later report in statistical terms. As a practicing psychiatrist over the past forty years I have seen a wide range of expressions of anxiety in citizens, from toddlers to the elderly. The incidence of anxiety appears to be increasing, and is expressed in many ways, both physically and emotionally.

For the past fifty years anxiety has been considered the reason for more than half the office visits to doctors. The anxiety may be about the person's health. The physical symptoms experienced also may be an expression of anxiety, as in tension headaches, irritable bowel syndrome, and many other tension states or stress-related conditions.

Another striking fact in recent decades has been the shift in incidence from infectious diseases to degenerative diseases, for several reasons, including life-style. Heart disease, arthritis, diabetes and cancer are common examples. This is true not only in the ever-increasing elderly population but also in younger persons. Breast cancer is epidemic, and will affect one out of nine women. This number is consistent for most of the industrialized nations of the world. Prostate cancer is occurring in younger men than in the past. Much of the media images of modern medicine focus on the technological advances with the implication that almost anything can be cured, and death kept at bay indefinitely. This obscures how much impairment and disability exist in chronic disease, for which modern medicine frequently has only limited answers. Where conventional medicine runs out of ideas or methods, often holistic or nonconventional methods may have an appeal, whether fully proven or not.

I do not wish to give the impression that anything with a label "holistic" is intrinsically good or safe. This is clearly not so, and some nonconventional methods can be not only useless but even dangerous, either by omission or commission. Each person must explore carefully before rushing into any treatment, whether conventional or nonconventional. There are no easy answers, especially as one explores outside the conventionally accepted approaches.

There is no lack of newspaper and magazine articles in the United States constantly reporting the rapidly increasing costs of medical care. The percent of Gross National Product has been rising every year, and is now beyond twelve percent. In addition the number of citizens who have no medical insurance or very limited coverage is also increasing. Most of the focus for possible solutions usually have been financial, with some suggestions for political and legislative solutions.

Few strong suggestions are raised to consider why so many people are apparently needing so much medical care in the first place. Mention is made of education and life-style factors, but medical skills are primarily for the diagnosis and treatment of disease, and there is little focus on prevention and health maintenance. It is ironic that most HMOs (Health Maintenance Organizations) offer diagnosis and medical treatment but give little attention to prevention. Not much energy, money or planning is devoted to true health maintenance. Again this is not a moral judgment, since conventional medical care does not have many tools or knowledge for primary prevention. This is not meant to be a criticism of conventional physicians, since they can only carry out what they have learned in their training and post-graduate education. I do not suggest that holistic medicine can offer complete answers either. Nevertheless, there is a distinct

interest by those physicians and nonmedical health practitioners who associate themselves with a holistic philosophy to encourage ways of maintaining and increasing
health and the avoidance of illness.

Six of the ten leading causes of death in the United States have a strong relationship
to life-style factors. Poor nutrition, the use of alcohol, lack of exercise, cigarette smoking, obesity, and stress are major ones. The most difficult challenge is to find ways that
can encourage people to do what is helpful and not to do the destructive actions that
lead to disease and death.

Holistic medicine clearly has stirred up controversy in the conservative circles of
medicine. Some practitioners have insisted that any suggestion that a person contributes
to their physical illness because of their personality makeup or emotional conflicts is a
monstrous idea. Any suggestion that a patient, particularly one with cancer, is anything
but a total victim is upsetting for some. This also is quickly misinterpreted repeatedly as
"blaming the victim." This is a distortion of what is being proposed. In fairness, however, to those who attack the inclusion of personality factors in physical disease, some
writings by holistic writers do read as if there were a tone of blame. Much heat can be
generated when one approaches the idea of mind/body unity. This is particularly so
when references are made to spiritual issues, such as meaning and purpose in illness.

It may appear as inevitable, or an occupational bias, that a psychiatrist declares that
mental and emotional factors play a significant part in any physical illness. I am not
alone in this view about mind/body unity. Even outside the field of clinical or behavioral psychology and psychiatry, there are many who are convinced that this is so.
Holistic medicine is not unique in this viewpoint, although it is clearly a major tenet of
it. When holistic medicine declares vigorously the unity of mind and body, and their
interaction with each other, then this can make a valuable contribution to health maintenance and healing.

George L. Engel, M.D., emeritus professor of medicine and psychiatry at the University of Rochester School of Medicine, wrote an article in *Science* in 1977 (Engel, 977).
The title was *The Need for a New Medical Model: a Challenge for Biomedicine*. Dr.
Engel declared that both the field of medicine and psychiatry adhered to a model of disease that was "no longer adequate for the scientific tasks and social responsibilities of
either medicine or psychiatry." He commented that medicine has focused only on
somatic or physical elements, excluding psychosocial issues. He also pointed to the
conflicts then within psychiatry, which was split between defining psychiatry as totally
outside the realm of medicine, or else only dealing with conditions that could be related
to brain dysfunction. The question Dr. Engel raised was whether the contemporary
model of disease was useful either for medicine or for psychiatry. He referred to the
prevailing model, which today is still essentially the same as in 1977, the biomedical
model of disease, one that has little room for social, psychological, and behavioral
dimensions of illness. This issue continues to be debated within the psychiatric profession. The 1991 president of the American Psychiatric Association raised this issue in
his presidential address, and specifically mentioned Dr. Engel's concept of "biopsychosocial medicine."

Dr. Engel further suggested that "in modern Western society biomedicine not only has provided a basis for the scientific study of disease, it has also become our own culturally specific perspective about disease, that is, our folk model." He further states that it has acquired the status of dogma, which then declares those who don't agree with it as heretics. He was urging a more inclusive scientific medical model that could benefit by looking at other societies and cultures, ancient and modern, preliterate and literate. "In all societies, the major criteria for identification of disease have always been behavioral, psychological, and social in nature."

Dr. Engel briefly reviewed the history of the mind/body dualism that was established in the sixteenth century, with the aid of Descartes and the church of the day. This fostered the idea of the body as a machine. This viewpoint was useful in that it allowed for the dissection of the body, no longer defined as the same as the soul. Disease was a breakdown of the machine, and a doctor's task was to repair the machine. As the more thoroughly scientific era of the nineteenth and twentieth centuries arrived, this produced remarkable achievements, but it put aside or dismissed mental/emotional and social factors.

To account for all illness requires more than a biochemical or biologic factor, and must include other dimensions, especially behavioral and psychosocial factors. Not to consider these, according to Dr. Engel, is to "bypass the patient's verbal account by placing greater reliance on technical procedures and laboratory measurements." Engel also looks at the doctor-patient relationship as vital to successful treatment. "The physician's role is, and always has been, very much that of educator and psychotherapist... These are outside the biomedical framework (Engel, 1977)."

Engel proposes a "biopsychosocial model that includes the patient as well as the illness." He also speaks of the physician as a healer in the new model that he proposes for physicians. He notes the inadequacies of the prevailing health care system. This includes the complaint that physicians are lacking in interest and understanding, "are preoccupied with procedures, and are insensitive to the personal problems of patients and families."

He describes the split within the psychiatric profession but points out that psychiatry is the only clinical discipline within medicine "concerned primarily with the study of man and the human condition." In the fifteen years since this article appeared, psychiatry has moved further from this more humanistic description and focused on biochemical and molecular science. It has lost some of the features leading to Dr. Engel's compliments. Nonetheless there is still some truth to his description. Since then the field of behavioral medicine, staffed almost entirely by psychologists and not physicians, has contributed to some of what Engel is calling for. He regrets that psychosomatic medicine has not had much impact, since the reductionistic and mechanistic demands of scientific methodologies are inappropriate for many of the problems to be studied. He also characterized medical schools as unreceptive or even hostile to exploration of psychosomatic phenomena. This may be changing a little with the development of psychoneuroimmunology.

Dr. Engel saw some hope for the future in the application of general systems theory as described by Von Bertalanffy, a biologist. Engel also spoke of a need to "develop holistic as well as reductionist explanations of life processes." He also hoped that his proposal of a new model might be expanded and absorbed in medical education. Thus the psychosocial dimensions of illness and health care would be taught and accepted by the younger generation of physicians. He concluded with saying that "the outcome will depend upon those who have the courage to try new paths and the wisdom to provide the necessary support."

Although Dr. Engel's ideas have not taken hold in any strong and obvious way in medical education, I remain optimistic that his insight will be justified and be increasingly applied. His writings and speeches have usually been presented within the mainstream of American medicine and its journals. Several years later he again presented his ideas in *The American Journal of Psychiatry* in "The Clinical Application of the Biopsychosocial Model." He again commented on the shortcomings of the biomedical model, and stated that: "The crippling flaw of the model is that it does not include the patient and his attributes as a person, a human being (Engel,1980)." He again emphasized the value of a systems view that sees each level of organization as part of a hierarchical or layered structure. Each level is part of a larger whole that in turn is part of a larger whole going up and down like a ladder. He is concerned to find a method that can combine science and humanism in actual practice, not just in theory.

Dr. Engel is proposing a different scientific model. As he says, "The hallmark of a scientific model is measured not by whether it is right or wrong but by how useful it is. It is modified or discarded when it no longer helps to generate and test new knowledge." He hopes to avoid dogmas that call upon tradition or authority for their influence. "Any dogma is in use when the basic principles of scientific method are ignored or avoided, whether it is 'biomedical science'" or what Engel calls counterdogmas, including "holistic" or "humanistic" medicine. When they "lean on faith and belief systems handed down from remote and obscure or charismatic authority figures, they tend to place science and humanism in opposition." He proposes that the biopsychosocial model can be used according to scientific principles, but different from what has been the biomedical model. In many respects he is suggesting much of what is part of the spirit of holistic medicine.

I have spoken of procedures and methods. Holistic medicine is as much an attitude to be implemented as it is any particular set of techniques. Several core principles associated with holistic medicine can be noted.

The uniqueness of the patient is a key concept. While this is acknowledged in orthodox medicine, it is easy to lose sight of this when treatment is in terms of a disease to be treated more than the patient as a person. Working in geriatric psychiatry I have seen a loss of focus on the individual sometimes. An elderly patient is given a medication in doses appropriate to a younger or middle-aged person, but far too strong for an eighty year old woman. Some of the scandals reported from time to time in newspapers about the excess use of sedative medications in nursing homes relate to this.

James Gordon, M.D. describes holistic medicine as including humanistic medicine, psychosomatic medicine, and behavioral medicine. Holistic medicine is becoming a gentle but persistent force in today's world as conventional medicine struggles against fragmentation, dehumanization and what Dr. Gordon calls "enforced passivity of human services—and indeed of life itself."

The total environment is part of a person's life, organism, illness and health. The spiritual dimension is also an issue when attitudes such as faith, hope and despair are under consideration. Holistic medicine can be more comfortable and interested than conventional medicine, in practices from other cultures outside the "mainstream," based on empirical—"what seems to work" as much as scientifically proven experiences. Some holistic physicians have included Chinese, Indian, Tibetan, and Native American practices. Acupuncture from Chinese medicine and herbal substances from Chinese, Indian, and Native American healing traditions are two examples.

In 1974 a thirty-three year old psychologist, Dr. Neil Fiore, discovered a small lump that was soon diagnosed as a cancer of the testicle. He had already developed a metastatic lesion in one lung. He wrote a forceful and explicit article about his entire fight to obtain a cure. His account was published in the *New England Journal of Medicine* in 1979 as "Fighting Cancer: One Patient's Perspective" (Fiore, 1979). He expanded the article later into a fuller guidebook for coping with the emotional aspects of cancer (Fiore, 1984). This book is one of an increasing number of excellent books available on coping with cancer and other serious or life-threatening illnesses.

Three years earlier Norman Cousins wrote *The Anatomy of an Illness,* published as an article and later as a book (Cousins, 1979). Both Dr. Fiore and Norman Cousins emphasize the need for patients to take a more active participation in their medical care. Dr. Fiore, after describing his involvement in some of the major decisions for treatment of his cancer, then makes several recommendations. In his shorter journal article he titled one section, "A Holistic Approach to the Patient with Cancer." Most of the suggestions are equally applicable to anyone with other serious diseases. He declared the need for both doctor and patient to acknowledge the importance of mind and emotions in the treatment. Not engaging them will mean "patient resistance to treatment, depression, and loss of will to live." Additional professionals are necessary besides the physician and nurse. Fiore insists "They (patients) need not act like helpless victims."

Medical social workers, psychologists and psychiatrists, health educators, and nutritionists are available in large hospitals, but Dr. Fiore comments that they are seldom called on to give cancer counseling. It would be useful if they would. Dr. Fiore also sees distinct value to patient support groups or individual psychotherapy. Stress management and changes in life-style are also critical needs to enhance conventional medical care.

I mention Dr. Fiore and his contributions as an example of a holistic approach that is broader than conventional medical care. More of what he has proposed is being brought into conventional treatment programs, but at a snail's pace. In a later chapter I shall describe support groups in some detail. In the following chapters I shall describe some of the procedures that are part of holistic medicine from a variety of traditions.

It is necessary to understand several legal issues that can affect the readiness of conventional physicians to adopt or permit themselves to explore practices included under holistic medicine. In most states in the United States, a reason cited in the statutes for the loss of a physician's license to practice is "unprofessional conduct." One of the definitions of unprofessional conduct in many states is the use of unproven methods, even if no harm was done to the patient, nor any complaint by a patient was registered.

The State of Alaska has passed a law, however, allowing a licensed Doctor of Medicine to use unproven methods, so long as no harm results, without this being considered unprofessional.

The State of Washington has a similar law before its legislature. Most states are not this liberal, and thus it is intimidating for conventional physicians to get ahead of the mainstream professional consensus. Despite this there are physicians who have accepted the risk and offer additional methods that are considered holistic, nonconventional or what the British have sometimes called "fringe medicine" (Inglis, 1965).

In recent years orthodox medical practitioners have supported the use of second opinions, and routinely obtain informed consent before starting any procedures or treatment that could have a risk to health or life. With less proven or nonconventional approaches it is no less true that there are risks. Individual decisions and individual responsibility are even more essential, when a person decides to go beyond "what the doctor orders." For many there may be too much anxiety connected with doing something that is not customary, familiar, or acceptable to the majority culture. For others there may be a need to seek some method in the hope that it will be more useful or supplement conventional methods. Sometimes it may be possible to blend or combine both the familiar and acceptable with the unproven, unknown and unfamiliar.

Some medical experts have estimated that eighty percent of all illnesses are self-limiting or will improve without any specific treatment. Ten percent need the application of modern technologically grounded medicine or surgery for relief and resolution. The remaining ten percent will worsen due to medical care. This last type of response is called "iatrogenic" or doctor-caused disease.

Part of the iatrogenic illness may be inevitable, and some is due to the consequences of hospitalization, and not directly due to the physician. A certain smaller part is due to incompetence. The obvious problem is that the patient cannot always judge from which type of illness he is suffering, and therefore does require diagnostic assistance and some form of treatment. Frequently, all that is required is reassurance that there is nothing serious. On the other hand immediate lifesaving surgery may be necessary. Hippocrates suggested something similar when he proposed that most healing occurs "vis medicatrix naturae"—by the healing way of Nature. It is difficult to believe this in today's world, with so many medications, diagnostic procedures, and medical specialties. I do not suggest we can get along without modern medicine's activities and contributions. There is room, still, for some alternative and complementary approaches that are non-conventional.

Surgery: Within the practice of conventional surgery, medicine and psychiatry, there is room for holistically oriented procedures that can enhance the effectiveness of scientifically-based practices. There now may be few surgeons who would call themselves holistic surgeons. I propose that it would be appropriate to use such a term whenever a surgical treatment includes some consideration of the patient as a whole person, and not just someone with a diseased organ.

Bernard Siegel, M.D. has been a practicing surgeon for more than twenty years in New Haven, Connecticut. He also founded an organization, ECaP, Exceptional Cancer

Patients, in 1978. The original purpose of the organization was to offer a support group for patients and former patients who were dealing with cancer. This became so successful that laypersons have been trained to be facilitators of similar groups throughout the United States and other countries. Dr. Siegel has also conducted workshops for patients, relatives and health professionals. He describes his ideas and methods in two excellent books, *Love, Medicine and Miracles* (Siegel, 1986) and *Peace, Love and Healing* (Siegel, 1989). I consider what he incorporated into his surgical practice as an example of holistic surgery.

Dr. Siegel gave an example of the use of drawings with surgical patients in a lecture I heard him present in 1985. He sometimes found it useful to have patients make simple drawings with colored crayons or pencils. Dr. Siegel had an eight years old boy with undescended testicle as a patient. Dr. Siegel asked the boy before surgery to draw a picture. The crucial question in such a physical problem is whether there is an intact testicle within the abdomen that had not descended during the child's development before birth, or the complete absence of a testicle. Sometimes nature has played a regrettable "trick" and in other cases, surgery can correct an unfinished process.

The boy drew a large airplane that he described as a bomber, also looking amazingly like a penis. Its two engines had a distinct resemblance to the scrotal sacs, with a testis in each. Dr. Siegel was reasonably sure that he would find the boy's condition repairable at surgery, based on the child's drawing, and his observations from many other patients' drawings. It is perhaps difficult to believe that the unconscious mind knows what is happening in the body. There is a large body of observations from many sources that supports this truth. This may seem rationally difficult to accept at first blush. This phenomenon of the body unconsciously revealing itself in drawings, in dreams, and on psychological tests, has been repeatedly documented. Several decades ago a psychologist, who was an expert on the use of the Rorschach ink blot test, could diagnosis patients with brain tumors from the results of the test. Dr. Gregg Furth describes the use of drawings, as Dr. Siegel reported, in detail in *Secret World of Drawings: Healing through Art* (Furth, 1988).

Another example of what I consider holistic elements in surgical treatment is the use of music in the operating-room. This has become increasingly common, even for surgeons who do not have any specific interest in holistic medicine. They have found that it is useful for both the operating-room staff and the patients. In one approach the patient herself brings a casette player with earphones into the operating-room with relaxing music or relaxation tapes. Some anesthesiologists have noticed that the patients are more relaxed with this practice.

In Dr. Siegel's writings he has advised surgeons to be conscious of what they say during an operation, though the patient is deeply anesthetized. Patients have reported having heard conversations while completely "under." Neurophysiologists who have studied brain-wave activity during anesthesia report that the brain centers for hearing show reactivity while the patient feels no pain and is not conscious in the ordinary sense.

When I underwent surgery for a thyroid tumor some years ago, I spoke with the anesthesiologist the night before surgery. I had written out a brief statement, an affirmation, on a three by five card. I asked him to say it to me several times during my operation, while I was anesthestized and unconscious. Although he was not familiar with this process, he was willing and cooperative. He already had a reputation for compassion, gentleness, and responsiveness to his patients' needs, so this was not too bizarre for him to agree to do. He didn't need to believe in what I asked of him, and I know he kept his promise. I had written on the card: "You, Henry, will have a rapid and uneventful recovery with a minimum of bleeding or discomfort, and without any complications."

The usual stay in the hospital for my particular procedure was four to five days. I left in three days with no problems associated with surgery. This does not prove anything at all, but it suggests what is possible. It allowed me to take an active part in my surgery, even while unconscious. It increased my comfort level with the anesthesiologist, whom I had known very slightly. I don't know if my being a physician made it easier to get cooperation or not. There are published reports by doctors who felt they did not necessarily receive better or even adequate care, when they were patients. The anxieties that doctors experience as patients are by no means less than the public's, and sometimes can be greater, since they know all the mistakes that might occur. An assertive layperson working in cooperation with their doctors also can obtain what they need to enhance their treatment.

Sometimes it may require that the patient speaks up without hesitation. I know of one example that is unusual but authentic. It is an example of spontaneous self-empowerment and self-responsibility. A woman had been given a diagnosis of cancer and was advised to undergo surgery. Although cancer often grows slowly before it reaches the stage of diagnosis, there is often a sense of urgency and even emergency created once the diagnosis is established. The patient often goes almost immediately to surgery. This had occurred for this woman. She was on the operating-room table within a week of her diagnosis of cancer. She still had many questions for her surgeon. She had liked him and trusted him. Before the start of the operation, she was conscious enough to ask the surgeon some questions. She also was experiencing a moderate amount of anxiety, and close to crying at moments. Her surgeon gently answered her questions.

The anesthesiologist, a male physician, was becoming annoyed with the slight delay in the schedule, and mentioned this to the surgeon. After a few more minutes of the patient speaking with the surgeon, the anesthesiologist said,

"Let's get this show on the road. We are running behind schedule." His tone of voice was one of irritation and coolness.

At this point he put his hands on the patient's arm. She experienced his touch as physically "ice cold." She then quickly told him to "get your f——g hands off of me," She then informed him, "You're fired!"

She requested that her surgeon get another anesthetist. The surgeon agreed to her request. The anesthesiologist left the operating room and another arrived about ten minutes later! This event is unusual and not typical of anesthesiologists, nor can any generalizations be made. Nonetheless, it is a vivid demonstration that patients do hire their physicians, and that a working partnership is desirable. Ordinarily, it does not nor should not require hostility or aggressiveness, only assertiveness. Desperation sometimes drives people to desperate measures. This woman's experience as a patient had been not only unholistic but unholy.

Holism in the practice of medicine and surgery cannot always include all the elements of mental/emotional, physical and spiritual considerations simultaneously. It may only be a combination of one element added to the usual practice. At other times it may include nonconventional, even unproven methods, that may work effectively in a particular patient. This happens often out of realistic desperation, because conventional methods may have offered very limited results. A remarkable account of one such experience in psychiatry is the story of Rickie.

Psychiatry: Rickie, when she was thirteen, developed an acute psychotic state that was thought to be a schizophrenic disorder. It was to last more than eleven years before significant improvement occurred. Her father is a psychiatrist who has described Rickie's struggles and his own as a father, husband, and professional in a highly readable book, *Rickie* (Flach, 1990), with recollections by Rickie herself, who is now forty. Dr. Frederic Flach's introductory note as the author states that he was strongly encouraged by others to tell the story to "help open minds toward new approaches to psychiatric care." He also declares "(our) experiences are not intended to detract from traditional methods nor be an endorsement of new, untested forms of therapy."

Never does he use the word nor suggest any connection to holistic medicine. I mention this account because Dr. Flach was willing to keep an open mind. This grew partly out of frustration and fear for the future of his daughter. Despite his professional adherence to scientific research and his skepticism of unproven methods, he was willing to explore other avenues.

It is not an easy path, after years of messages from professors, textbooks and medical journals, for most physicians to tolerate or accept the unproven. Six years before the breakthrough that led to her improvement her mother had asked Rickie's psychiatrist several times about orthomolecular therapy. It is a controversial method of treating psychosis with minerals, vitamins and other nutritional substances. Reports of research by Canadian and American psychiatrists had apparently disproved the theory behind orthomolecular treatment.

Rickie's psychiatrist urged her father, Dr. Flach, to dissuade the mother of any such ideas. Simultaneously mother was urging Dr. Flach to press for orthomolcular therapy for their daughter, who had been ill at that point for more than four years, with little to no improvement.

Dr. Flach comments in the book that he knew "it would never be implemented at W. (Rickie's current hospital), and having learned from colleagues familiar with it that orthomolecular therapy was held in general disrepute, verging on charlatanism, I did not."

Six years later, after several more hospitalizations with no progress, Dr. Flach did seek orthomolecular evaluation and treatment for his daughter. While attending a medical school reunion Dr. Flach met a classmate who was well-acquainted with a major center where research and use of orthomolecular medicine was available. After hearing praise for this approach, he said to his classmate, "I'm sure you know the mere mention of nutritional therapy makes a lot of psychiatrists see red." His classmate acknowledged this was so.

"Do you think it really works," Dr. Flach asked, with more than professional curiosity.

"In some cases dramatically. It's not just vitamins. It's a total nutritional play. Pfeiffer [Carl Pfeiffer, M. D., founder of the Princeton Bio Center] analyzes mineral, histamine levels, other factors too and chooses a regimen according to his lab findings."

About the same time Dr. Flach heard this, he also received another suggestion that was unorthodox. This, too, would eventually contribute to Rickie's later recovery. Dr. Flach earlier had met a film producer with whom he participated in creating a teaching film on depression. As he describes it, he felt very comfortable with this man so that he eventually shared his anxieties about Rickie.

The film producer responded with an unusual suggestion. He described a former neighbor who was an optometrist who had studied at the Gesell Institute in New Haven, Connecticut. This is an institute that has engaged in the study of childhood development for several decades, but in recent years has included research and training in developmental optometry. This is a special field within optometry that had developed a variety of techniques for examining children's vision from a much wider range of approach than traditional optics. One feature of developmental optometry, later called behavioral optometry, is visual training. It is used, for example, for children and adults with perceptual difficulties, dyslexia and other learning problems. The film producer urged Dr. Flach to contact his former neighbor, the developmental optometrist, and get an evaluation of Rickie, who was now twenty-three.

"You just don't know what might turn up." Dr. Flach attempted to encourage Rickie's psychiatrist to explore this direction. Similar to his experience with suggesting orthomolecular treatment, he received highly negative reactions to his request for a specialized optometric evaluation. After making several requests that were met with polite skepticism, Dr. Flach received a final dismissal of his proposals. As he reports his experience (Flach, 1990):

"Finally, he dismissed my idea altogether, saying that he had discussed the matter with a local ophthalmologist, [M. D.] who found the notion completely absurd."

It was not too long after this that Rickie's psychiatrist informed the family that he could no longer agree to treat her, since there had been no progress at all. He recommended that it would be better if she were placed in a state hospital. The implication was she could remain there for the rest of her life.

This was now ten years since her initial episode of "breakdown." Dr. Flach then arranged for the optometric evaluation with Dr. Melvin Kaplan, a developmental optometrist. Also an orthomolecular evaluation at the Princeton Bio Center was scheduled for his daughter. He told Rickie, he reports (Flach, 1990):

"This isn't easy for me. It means going against everything I've ever been taught, and I can't promise it will work. My colleagues scoff at Pfeiffer's work."

Both the optometric and the orthomolecular examinations did show unusual findings, followed up by specific and effective treatments. I shall not attempt to summarize any further the unfolding of Rickie's cure and rehabilitation. I encourage anyone interested to read Dr. Flach and Rickie's report of her trials and tribulations, as well those of her family's. The book does not claim to be a complete answer to mental illness, but it does demonstrate several holistic principles, including openmindedness and a tolerance for the unproven in the face of the unknown.

Internal Medicine: An example of conventional medical practice that incorporates many holistic principles and practices is the program for the treatment of coronary heart disease developed by Dean Ornish, M.D. His research and treatment program are based on carefully designed scientific methods. It is still not yet the most commonly used approach compared to the use of coronary bypass surgery and medications. Dr. Ornish does not at any point use the term nor refer to holistic medicine. At the same time he writes in his introduction to *Dr. Dean Ornish's Program for Reversing Heart Disease* (Ornish, 1990), "This is a book about healing your heart: physically, emotionally, and spiritually. The Opening Your Heart program described in this book can help transform your life." The subtitle of his book is "The Only System Scientifically Proven to reverse Heart Disease Without Drugs or Surgery." He has been able to demonstrate clearly a partial reversal of coronary artery blockage through a program of nutrition, exercise, yoga, meditation, and group support. He also shares in detail his past personal struggles as a human being. I consider his contribution a fine example of a holistic approach to medical care. It exemplifies the full appreciation of mind/body unity besides touching on the place of spirituality in health and illness. The heart that breaks emotionally also can break physically.

It is proper next to look at some wider dimensions of health and illness care not usually included in conventional medicine. Closest to orthodox medicine is Osteopathy or osteopathic medicine. Usually, it is indistinguishable from what a doctor of medicine practices. There are, however, some twists that are not familiar to patients who only consult a conventional physician.

3

Osteopathic Medicine

When I was in medical school I never heard anyone mention osteopathy or osteopathic medicine. Neither was I aware of any osteopathic physicians in practice. I don't recall if there was any acknowledgment there was such a degree as D.O., Doctor of Osteopathy. Although I belonged to the History of Medicine Club, I didn't learn about the struggles during the nineteenth century between conventional medicine and osteopathic medicine. Conventional medical education did not encourage any explorations outside the narrow confines of scientific medicine.

The founder of osteopathic medicine was Andrew Taylor Still. He was the son of a frontier Methodist preacher or circuit rider who also was a country physician. Besides learning from his father as an apprentice in medicine, Andrew Still also studied at the Kansas City School of Physicians and Surgeons.

After several years in practice as a conventional physician in Kirksville, Missouri, Dr. Still lost three of his children in one year, because of spinal meningitis. He became profoundly upset with the shortcomings of his profession. This led him to spend the next ten years searching for a better approach to health and illness.

In 1874 he formulated his principles of osteopathy in which he declared that the body has its own innate capacities for healing. He also declared that the structure of the body affects its various functions. He meant by this that the shape and position of the skeletal structure were central to maintaining health. He found that the correction of posture problems, mobilization of joints, and alignment of the spine improved health and aided in the healing of disease. This was a revival of an ancient Hippocratic principle that the body can heal itself with proper assistance, preferably without any drugs.

When he opened his practice in Kirksville, Missouri, he became famous for his ability to help patients. By 1892 he had organized and opened the first college of osteopathy. His ideas and methods were different from the mainstream thinking of his medical colleagues who considered him an eccentric at first. Like many innovators he was attacked and criticized.

When he established the American School of Osteopathy, the policy of the school was to permit admission to women and Afro-Americans. This was in contrast to almost all the conventional medical schools of that era. As he became more well-known, not only conventional physicians attacked osteopathy, but also homeopathic physicians joined forces to attack osteopathy. Ironically homeopathic physicians in earlier decades experienced intense attacks and criticism by conventional physicians.

Still was a deeply religious man, and believed that healing was an innate God-given capacity of the human body. The charter of his school permitted the granting of the M.D. degree, but Still proposed the D.O. degree for the physicians who graduated from his school. Thus the graduates were called Doctors of Osteopathy, or osteopathic physicians.

One of Still's students, John Martin Littlejohn, originally from Scotland, established the second osteopathic school in the United States in Chicago. He later returned to the British Isles. He then established the British School of Osteopathy in England in 1917. By 1917 there were five thousand osteopathic physicians in the United States and abroad.

At present there are thirty thousand osteopathic physicians in the United States. All fifty states license osteopathic physicians. They have essentially the same rights as Doctors of Medicine. The training now for osteopathic physicians in the United State is a four-year program after at least three years of undergraduate college. (During World War II all pre-medical students including myself went to medical school after three years of college). Besides what is included in conventional medical education, the osteopathic physician-in-training learns manipulative procedures derived from Dr. Still's principles.

The distinction between M.D.s and D.O.s in the United States today is often small, since many D.O.s do not apply their manipulation and touch techniques. Most graduates of osteopathic colleges become family practitioners, often practicing in rural areas, but there are osteopathic physicians who are specialists in all the same fields as M.D.s. This includes surgery, psychiatry, and neurology for example.

The philosophy and spirit of osteopathy can be considered as contributing to a holistically-oriented system of medicine. Some osteopaths accept with conviction Dr. Still's original views about the healing power of Nature. They may be more attentive to the whole person than is sometimes true for conventional medicine. Because osteopathy includes physical manipulation of the body, this should not obscure the fact that Still's philosophy was equally concerned with the inherent healing processes of the body as well. In a textbook, *The Principles of Osteopathy*, its author, Leon E. Page, D.O., comments:

> No form of therapy can be considered curative in itself. The final restoration of physiological balance is brought about by powers within the body many of which are as yet little understood. It should always be remembered that the duty of the physician is not to cure

disease but rather to create conditions that will be most favorable for the operation of defensive mechanisms of the body.

Dr. Page quotes a well-known saying of Andrew Still, "the rule of the artery is supreme." By this he meant that not only the blood but all body fluids "are the agents for ultimate recovery of tissue after disease or injury, whether by immunity, tissue repair or regeneration." Andrew Still developed many physical maneuvers to encourage healing, but did not himself develop a fixed set of manipulations that were always to be applied in the same way.

Among the several types of osteopathic manipulative treatments commonly used are soft tissue methods, passive movement techniques, and "high velocity thrusts." Several decades ago I had my first personal encounter as a patient of an osteopathic physician in Connecticut. Someone had suggested him to me when I mentioned I was experiencing shoulder pain.

After he took my history and examined me, he performed several maneuvers with my arm and shoulder. He also massaged and rubbed my shoulder. It felt "good." I was conscious of the difference between this experience and all previous conventional medical examinations and treatments. The physical touch immediately brought to mind the phrase, "the laying on of hands." He also prescribed several simple exercises for my shoulder that I was to do at home. I saw him two or three more times and no longer experienced any problem after that.

My training as a conventional physician included techniques of physical diagnosis, such as tapping on chests and abdomens, and knowing where to probe here and there carefully to feel for enlarged organs, such as the spleen and liver. Still, there was no message about touching in a consciously healing way. Scientific medicine has had little to say about the "healing energy of touch." Generations of mothers and registered nurses know more about this than most conventional physicians.

Since only five percent of American physicians are osteopaths, only a few citizens can be treated by them. Although I had been able to consult an osteopathic physician in Hartford, Connecticut, I had not otherwise been aware of any others during my twenty-nine years in Connecticut. Since living in Maine, I am now far more aware of osteopathic physicians. There are several osteopathic hospitals in the state, an osteopathic medical school, and at least three osteopathic physicians in my own community of nine thousand.

William Garner Sutherland, a student of Still, developed osteopathy in the cranial field. His studies led him to the understanding that the sutures, or joints, of the skull where the various bones come together were important, and capable of very slight movements. Sutherland spent thirty years developing his ideas and findings into a diagnostic and treatment program. Derivatives of his work are sometimes called cranio-sacral therapy, when practiced by other non-osteopathic health professionals. As explained by Stephen Sandler, D.O. in his book, *Osteopathy, the Illustrated Guide* (Sandler, 1989):

Inside the skull, the brain is suspended by sheets of fascial tissue known as the meninges, that are held in tension by their bony attachments. The meninges extend all the way down the vertebral column to the sacrum at the base of the spine. This linkage provides a system called a reciprocal tension mechanism, which connects the movement of the skull bones and the movement of the sacrum. The fascia is attached at one end in the skull and at the other in the pelvis.

Osteopaths who have studied and specialized in this system maintain that palpation on the skull and sacrum can pick up a rhythmic pulsation distinct from the respiratory rhythm or heartbeat and pulse of the blood. This pulsation is the reverberation of the cerebrospinal fluid, which bathes both the brain and the spinal cord.

The principles of osteopathy in the cranial field are based on the viewpoint that disturbances in the normal cranial bones' movements cause a disturbance of the cranial rhythm described by Dr. Sandler. Gently guiding and releasing the tensions through very mild pressure on the different cranial bone near the sutures of the skull, where one bone lies next to another, can lead to diagnosis and treatment of a variety of disorders in a gentle non-invasive way.

In some osteopathic hospitals osteopathic treatment in the cranial field is given to newborns at birth. This is to correct some of the deformities of the skull that occur in difficult or prolonged labor and birth. Children also respond well to the gentle approach that osteopathic treatment in the cranial field offers. Dr. Sandler also describes the value of these procedures for infants and very young children with colic, strabismus (eye squint), disturbed sleep or constant crying.

In England and Europe the practice of osteopathy is different. Osteopaths are not defined as physicians and do not have the same legal status as in the U.S. Osteopathy still ranks as a major complementary therapy to conventional medicine. A regular M. D. in England may refer to a registered osteopath. There is no official licensing. Anyone may call themselves an osteopath. There is at the same time, a Register of osteopaths. British osteopaths practice manipulative therapy based on Still's principles, but do not claim to be offering a complete alternative form of medicine. They do not practice any surgery or obstetrics, nor does their training include any pharmacology or drug prescription.

In France and Belgium regulations require osteopaths first to be trained as physiotherapists. They also spend four years in weekend training programs learning osteopathic diagnosis, principles and techniques. This is followed by an examination which leads to a Certificate in Osteopathy.

In Australia a program began in Melbourne in 1987, based on the British School of Osteopathy for the training of osteopaths. Eventually there will be graduates who will establish their own register of practitioners.

One of Andrew Still's students in the 1880s was a Canadian-born grocer, Daniel David Palmer, who settled in Davenport, Iowa. According to some accounts, he did not finish his training due to disagreements with his teacher. He also was a practitioner of "magnetic healing," a form of hypnosis. In 1895 he became the founder of chiropractic.

4

Chiropractic

On September 18, 1895 Daniel David Palmer did some spinal manipulations on his janitor, Harvey Lillard. Following the manipulation Lillard regained his hearing after seventeen years of deafness. Understandably Palmer felt convinced that the theory he had developed was correct. He believed that all illness was related to disturbances of spinal misalignment. Thus was born the practice of modern chiropractic. "Chiro" is the Greek word for "hand" and "praktikor" means "done by." The ancient Greeks, Romans, and Chinese had done "bone-setting" for centuries. Bone-setters worked throughout the history of Europe, separate from the medical profession. Hippocrates, father of modern medicine, said, "Look well to the spine, for many diseases have their origin in the dislocations of the vertebral column."

At one point in his unfolding career Palmer was arrested for practicing medicine without a license, although he was not using methods that were part of conventional medicine. Palmer believed in a "Universal Intelligence" in all living matter that was responsible for not only life itself but also for survival and growth. He saw the nervous system and the brain as the central source for control of the body that then determined the health of the body. He believed that interference of nerve impulses from the brain through the spinal column would result in disease. The interference was due to mechanical pressure by spinal bones when a "subluxation," or slight dislocation, was present. In recent years a number of journals and organizations have reported clinically proven effectiveness. The Rand Corporation, a prestigious research organization, reported in July of 1991 on a study of effectiveness, and also several Worker's Compensation Review Boards. A 1990 issue of the *British Medical Journal* also gave positive comments. Palmer's theory of "single cause, single treatment" has not been satisfactorily accepted or tolerated by all conventional medical doctors. Nonetheless, many citizens throughout the United States and Europe have accepted chiropractic treatment for relief of some ailments.

Palmer founded a college of chiropractic in 1897. His son, B. J. Palmer, later took over the school and became a highly successful practitioner, teacher and businessman. While all chiropractors agree that the subluxation plays a role in disease and structural malfunction, opinions differ in defining proper treatment. Traditional approaches use spinal adjustments only, while more liberal practitioners use other methods, such as nutritional counseling, physical therapy and exercise therapy.

Chiropractors usually restrict their manipulations mainly to the spine. Osteopathic procedures, on the other hand, may include different joints throughout the body. The most common problems for which people seek chiropractic treatment are back and neck problems. The public consults chiropractors for back related symptoms three times more often than all other types of physicians, according to a *New York Times* nationwide poll. Chiropractors also report excellent results for headaches.

Due to legal restraints the American Medical Association does not any longer actively discourage or forbid orthodox or conventional physicians from referring to chiropractors or other nonconventional practitioners. Nonetheless most M.D.s are still critical and cautious about chiropractic treatment, because of its lack of a scientifically-based theory. I would hazard a guess that few M.D.s have ever experienced any chiropractic treatment personally. It is also common for many patients of conventional physicians not to share with their doctor that they have also consulted and received treatment from a chiropractor. I do not recall that I have ever mentioned this to my family physician. I have obtained chiropractic treatments both in Connecticut and in Maine, where I have lived for the past eight years. One type of chiropractic treatment can be considered preventive maintenance, in which a person has monthly treatments for the back or neck, to prevent the return of bothersome symptoms, such as pain or stiffness.

Since the early 1970s there have been several studies that support the value of chiropractic. As reported by Richard Wild in his article on chiropractic in *Hands-On Healing* (Feltman,1989):

> The Oregon Workmen's Compensation Board found that chiropractors got workers with back injuries back on the job faster than [M.D.] physicians did. Of those chiropractic patients studied, 82% returned to work within one week of their injury; of those patients who sought a physician's care, only 41% returned within a week.

Wild also refers to a study at the University of Utah that reviewed two hundred and thirty-two persons, some of whom had been treated for back problems by medical doctors and some by chiropractors. Wild states: "The researchers concluded that the intervention of a chiropractor in problems [related to] neck and spine injuries was at least as effective as that of a physician."

Earlier I mentioned hearing a chiropractor lecture at a conference on Comparative Systems of Healing. At one point in the conference each speaker met with a small group of participants. I attended the one led by the chiropractor. He asked for a volunteer to demonstrate some chiropractic techniques. I volunteered, without any specific problem or goal other than to experience the procedure. I was willing to stick my neck out.

I came forward and sat on a low stool in front of the small audience. He then proceeded to carry out a common chiropractic maneuver with my head and neck. He asked me to relax my head as best as I could. He then lifted my head slightly and leaned it to one side. He then gave it a twist and a slight jerk. I heard a cracking sound. He then repeated the procedure on the other side. Again I could hear a cracking noise.

I then sat up straight and moved my head slowly from side to side, partly to assure myself that it was still attached to my body. It obviously was. I then realized that I could move it more freely from shoulder to shoulder, possibly ten or fifteen degrees wider in each direction.

I quickly recalled that I had a minor problem with my neck fourteen years earlier while in the Air Force, stationed in Alaska. I had experienced an acute pain in my right neck for about a week. X-rays then showed some early signs of osteoarthritis, with calcium deposits on several vertebrae in my neck. I was told to use some aspirin and "just live with it," since there was no specific treatment for it.

Over the next decade and a half I would occasionally experience twinges in my upper shoulders. This was due to pressure on the nerve roots as they exited from the spinal column and traveled through the neck vertebrae's openings. The chiropractic adjustment apparently "unjammed" my neck and allowed more movement. I do not recall whether the restriction gradually came back or not. My recollection is that it did not. I did not have any more acute problems with my neck for the next nineteen years until 1986. Yet, I do not choose to give all the credit to this one chiropractic maneuver. Several years later I did undertake a few chiropractic adjustments from time to time. I also underwent several years of bioenergetic therapy, a body-oriented psychotherapy that involves much work with muscular tensions, breathing, and emotional release, along with verbal psychotherapy. My posture definitely improved because of Bioenergetic therapy. The improvement in my posture created less strain on my neck. I also was less quick to allow some of my life's experiences to be a pain in the neck emotionally.

I did have another acute flare-up of right neck pain, thirty-three years after my Alaska experience. I have described the details of this in the first chapter. The circumstance of consulting a physician led to the discovery of a thyroid tumor. I consider the arthritis on the right side a gift, since I had not felt any symptoms of any kind to suggest the presence of a thyroid tumor. Even a pain in the neck can turn into a gift. I subsequently did also undertake some monthly chiropractic treatments. My neck has not produced any unpleasant symptoms, such as pain, in the following six years.

Applied Kinesiology: In 1964 Dr. George Goodheart of Detroit, Michigan created a new form of chiropractic, which he called Applied Kinesiology. He discovered that testing the strength of individual muscles showed a correlation with internal organ disturbances. He also noticed that most muscle pairs from one side of the body to the other would frequently have one set tight and the other set weak. This would cause a pulling on one side more than the other. The same would hold true for sets of muscles on the front and back of the body.

Instead of seeking to relax the excessively tight muscles, he developed methods for strengthening the weak muscles. He also integrated some concepts and methods of an osteopathic physician, Dr. Frank Chapman, who lived in the early 1900s. Chapman had discovered lymphatic reflexes that could be massaged or rubbed to improve body functioning. Dr. Goodheart also integrated some principles and methods from Chinese medicine as well, including attention to the energy pathways called *meridians*. What gradually evolved into Applied Kinesiology was a system for examining the body with the use of the body to detect early signs of dysfunction. The dysfunctions were not only physical ones but also biochemical and emotional ones. Dr. Goodheart developed a more holistic approach to chiropractic treatment than the classic approach, and far more extensive than had been true for the more liberal "Mixers."

One major problem that Applied Kinesiology presents is that a major feature of it, muscle-testing, requires careful and sensitive application to prevent "operator influence." This can sometimes produce results that the examiner was anticipating, a self-fulfilling expectation. Andrew Weil, M. D. in *Health and Healing* (Weil, 1983) expresses total skepticism about Applied Kinesiology. He is cautious in stating that he cannot make a definite judgment about it. He does admit that the technique possibly does reveal information about the body. Simultaneously he suggests that the results could be "a parlor trick" and that some holistic practitioners have accepted it too un-critically. I can fully appreciate this reaction since some of its techniques produce star-tling results. It also is often used without sufficient and extensive training. I am more familiar with it than most citizens and physicians. I undertook the one-hundred-hour ten month training course given by the International College of Applied Kinesiology in 1977.

Most of the thirty students in the program were chiropractors, except myself and one dentist. The material was unfamiliar not only to me but also to the chiropractors as well. Since then there have been applications of Applied Kinesiology outside the field of chiropractic. I knew a psychologist who has used AK (Applied Kinesiology) in her practice of psychotherapy. She would muscle-test before and after a counseling session. She would test the strength or weakness of certain muscles to evaluate the emotional intensity of a particular topic the patient was discussing.

It is not apparent how one can make sense of the connections that are shown between body processes, particularly muscles, and mental and emotional states. I have person-ally observed examples of this being demonstrated in which suggestion or operator influence were not strong influences.

John Diamond, M. D., trained in Australia and practicing in the United States, has made extensive use of Applied Kinesiology in his psychiatric practice. He has devel-oped a form of AK he calls BK, or *Behavioral Kinesiology*. He has shown, with this technique, the influence or environmental elements on the body, including music, nutri-tion, and clothes.

His first book, *Behavioral Kinesiology* (Diamond, 1979) also placed emphasis on the role of the thymus gland, previously considered in conventional medicine as of little importance. In the past ten years, however, newer research has shown the thymus gland is of greater importance than previously suspected (Wisneski, 1990).

Dr. Diamond expanded his use of behavioral kinesiology to include a means of con-necting the muscle-testing system of Applied Kinesiology with the energy meridians of Chinese medicine, which in turn are associated with emotional states. He describes this process in *Life Energy* (Diamond, 1985). The teachers of Applied Kinesiology who are chiropractors find Diamond's work too great a departure from Dr. George Goodheart's original contributions to be considered "standard procedure." Only further research and application will decide if AK and BK are as valuable and useful as Dr. Goodheart claims. From my personal experiences hearing Dr. Goodheart speak and demonstrate his methods, I think there is evidence that AK can make a contribution to health maintenance and enhancement.

Now only a minority of chiropractors have been trained to use Applied Kinesiology in their practice. It does allow for a much broader scope of diagnosis and treatment than usual. This has carried the practice of chiropractic well beyond Palmer's original form of chiropractic treatment, offering solutions for a wider range of health problems than traditional chiropractic. It does not usually match the wider scope of treatment that is included in Naturopathy, as practiced by naturopathic physicians. Naturopathic physicians are trained to use manipulative techniques similar to osteopathic and chiropractic ones, but they also use homeopathy, herbal medicine, and several other approaches.

Both osteopathy and chiropractic developed in the United States in the late nineteenth century as departures from conventional medical theory and practice. Osteopathy as currently practiced in the United States often cannot be distinguished from conventional medical practice, unless manipulative treatment is used. Chiropractic is clearly outside the realms of conventional medicine, as defined by conventional or orthodox physicians.

5

Homeopathy

A German physician, Samuel Hahnemann, M. D., was the founder of homeopathy. He was born in 1755 and died in 1843. Hahnemann published his major text, *Organum of Medicine* in 1810. In 1880 his worldwide reputation made him an outstanding hero in medicine. Several hospitals still bear his name. Very few citizens or physicians today are familiar with his name. Dr. Hahnemannn, like Andrew Still, had lost faith in the methods that he had learned in medical school and were the common practices of his day. This was the era in the history of medicine called *The Heroic Age of medicine*. The methods of treatment were heroic and drastic. These included blood-letting and purging with strong substances, such as mercury salts. Unfortunately mercury was poisonous when given in the recommended doses. The "proof" that the mercury was taking effect included the production of excessive saliva, an early sign of mercury poisoning.

George Washington probably died as much from his bloodletting treatment as from his terminal illness. Hahnemann was less enthusiastic about such measures, and recommended supportive measures such as exercise, fresh air and good food. Hahnemann was also a religious and spiritual man, believing that healing came from God and Nature. He believed there was a life force that animated the body. He called it the "vital force." Hahnemann was also an accomplished translator who read medical texts in other languages. A chief spokesmen for the heroic method then was a professor of medicine at the University of Edinburgh, Dr. William Cullen. When Hahnemann translated Cullen's *Materia Medica* he found little evidence that experimental findings were the basis for recommended prescriptions. There appeared to be no logical reason for their use. Hahnemann came to try out substances on himself and establish "provings" as he called them. Andrew Weil has pointed out (Weil, 1988) that Hahnemann "is never given credit for it, (but) he is really the father of experimental pharmacology, and pharmacologists today might still benefit from reading his suggestions."

Hahnemann noticed that the people who were surviving the malaria epidemics in

Europe were the ones that were taking cinchona bark, from which quinine was later derived. As an experiment Hahnemann took four drams (0.5 ounces) of cinchona twice daily, and soon developed the intermittent fevers that are characteristic of malaria. This was Hahnemann's first "proving" of a substance that might be used as a medicinal preparation. He studied the properties of other substances that might be of use as medicines by observing their effects on healthy humans. Hahnemann studied more than ninety medicines in his lifetime by performing provings on himself, his family and his friends.

He gradually developed a new system of medicine he called homeopathy. The word refers to a system of medical treatment based on the use of minute quantities of remedies that in massive doses produce effects similar to those of the disease being treated. The phrase, like cures like, is an essential tenet of homeopathy. The opposite approach of conventional medicine was called *allopathy*, meaning "fighting against disease." The word, *antibiotic*, literally means "against the life" of the bacteria. Fevers are treated with substances in conventional medicine to counteract and fight the fever.

Homeopathy is an empirical science. It is based on what has been observed repeatedly to be true. For example, the homeopathic preparation of Arnica Montana is observed objectively and subjectively to heal soft tissue trauma. It has also been seen that Arnica can cause such trauma, such as easy bruising, aching, and soreness if taken repeatedly over time.

Another strange phenomenon that Hahnemann discovered and then developed as part of his treatment system was the use of increasingly dilute amounts of medicines. He felt convinced they could act more powerfully than less dilute ones. He applied his religious orientation to his work and believed that the spirit was more important than material reality. Therefore, a highly dilute substance could be seen as containing the essence or spirit of a substance even if the amount of material was so small there were no more molecules in the diluted solution. He called this the *Law of Infinitesimals*. The process of dilution that produced a more powerful result was called "potentialization" of a substance.

The potency or strength worked in a reverse direction. The greater the potentialization, or dilution, the more powerful was the effect of one dose of the medicine. Hahnemann and other homeopathic physicians found that smaller potencies must be repeated but one dose of a high potency (highly dilute) may be all that is necessary to bring about cure. This is the experience in modern-day homeopathic practice.

Hahnemann's original form of treatment used only a single substance as the cure for an ailment, and never used two simultaneously. If the first one didn't produce results, then a second one could be considered but not to be given at the same time. Hahnemann developed other rules and laws of treatment, which became part of his original system. His homeopathic system of treatment became well-established and famous throughout Europe by the time he died at eighty-eight in 1843.

Homeopathy became a part of American medicine in 1828. Constantine Hering established the first homeopathic medical school in 1835 in Allentown, Pennsylvania. This later moved to Philadelphia and became the Hahnemann Medical College and Hospital, still in existence but no longer homeopathic.

Constantine Hering was a prestigious American homeopath. He is well-known for a proving he did with the venom of the South American Bushmaster snake. He and his wife went to South America to capture one of these snakes, and returned to the United States with its venom. He accidentally touched the venom with his bare hands. Soon he proceeded to have extraordinary hallucinations, fevers, and other unusual symptoms. When his sickness passed, the first words he said to his wife were, "Did you note the symptoms?"

His wife, well-versed in homeopathy, had indeed written down all of her husband's strange and vivid symptoms. Today the homeopathic remedy, Lachesis, derived from the Bushmaster snake's venom, is often used for the treatment of individuals with severe problems such as psychosis, and also for less pathological symptoms such as hypertension and menopausal hot flashes. A popular layperson's guide to homeopathic medicines (Cummings & Ullman, 1984) lists Lachesis as one of thirty remedies recommended in a home remedy kit among one hundred common homeopathic remedies.

Homeopathy became increasingly popular in the United States during a period when conventional medicine was under heavy attack. This occurred in the first half of the nineteenth century, during the Popular Health Movement that encouraged citizens to take more active responsibility for their health. Licensing laws for physicians were abolished in many states for a time. Anyone who defined themselves as qualified could practice any form of healing they wished.

In 1846, during this period of extreme liberalism, the conventional physicians organized the American Medical Association to combat homeopathic physicians. Conventional physicians were forbidden to refer to homeopathic physicians.

Homeopathy gradually became involved in dissension within its ranks. A split occurred among homeopathic physicians, between a small minority who remained loyal to Hahnemann's principles and used only one remedy at a time, and the majority who included some allopathic remedies in larger doses. They also consulted with allopathic physicians as well. Many homeopathic physicians gradually became more completely allopathic.

According to Andrew Weil (Weil, 1988), by 1900 there were about fifteen thousand homeopathic physicians in the United States, a sixth of all M. D.s. There were then twenty-two homeopathic medical colleges. By 1923 only two were still operating, and they eventually closed or changed over to conventional medical education. Few Americans are familiar today with homeopathy, although in the past twenty years there has been a revival of interest. India presently has the largest number of homeopathic practitioners. Germany and France are also far more familiar with it than in the U. S.

Members of the British royal family are the patrons of homeopathic hospitals in England, and have consulted homeopathic physicians for several generations, since the 1830s. Homeopathy is sometimes called "The Royal Medicine." When I was in London in 1987 I walked past a very large, impressive-looking building near Russell Square. It was the Royal London Homeopathic Hospital on Great Ormond St. Pharmacies in France and Germany sell many homeopathic substances. Some of the largest homeopathic pharmaceutical companies are in Germany and France.

To a Western scientist homeopathy does not "make sense" since it does not follow the accepted principles of chemistry and medicine. Some critics would insist that it is all a matter of suggestion, if not outrageous nonsense. For those citizens who find it a source of relief and cure, it is nonetheless highly appreciated.

One possible explanation for why homeopathic remedies work has been a theory based on electromagnetic activity. Supporting this is the usual present-day recommendation that anyone taking homeopathic remedies should not use an electric blanket, since it interferes with effectiveness. Also certain strong odors such as menthol and camphor also destroy the healing effects of homeopathic remedies. Certain other substances, coffee for example, inhibit the effects of a homeopathic remedy.

A highly prestigious scientific journal, *Nature*, published an article in 1988 by a French scientist of international reputation. Jacques Beneviste described an experiment that appeared to give clear proof of the homeopathic principle that a very high dilution could still have a biological effect on cells. The dilution was so large there were no molecules of the original substance remaining, but the diluted liquid still had an antibody effect on white blood cells.

The exact title of the article in *Nature* was "Human basophil degranulation triggered by very dilute antiserum against IgE." As described in Prescriber (Volume V, number 4), newsletter published by the BOIRON Educational Institute, a division of a large homeopathic pharmaceutical company:

> One of the members of his research team did an experiment "on the side" with homeopathically dilute substances. When the subordinate showed his results to Beneviste, Beneviste didn't believe them. To prove the researcher wrong, Beneviste repeated the experiment. To his astonishment, the homeopathically diluted substances did have measurable effects on the cells. After years of more experiments, repeated in laboratories in Israel, Italy and Canada, Beneviste and his colleagues succeeded in having their report published in *Nature*. As a result of the [disbelief] of the committee who reviewed the paper, *Nature* sent three men intent on investigating the presumed fraud (none were experts in the field of research) to Beneviste's lab.

One of the investigators was a professional magician, Randi. He joined the other two non-researchers to declare that the study was questionable because of sloppiness in the research. *Nature* then issued a retraction of the article. A further accounting of the "Beneviste Affair" is described in *Prescriber:*

> Beneviste reacted angrily and noted that no other research done in his lab had ever been subjected to such unfair treatment. Under orders from his superior in France, Beneviste withdrew from the public eye for 18 months, while continuing to pursue his research. He has now broken his silence with an article in a scientific journal reporting further research.
>
> His team has found that homeopathic substances lose their effectiveness if exposed to a magnetic field—which lends support to Beneviste's theory that the potency of homeopathic substances reside in their electromagnetic field, not in the presence or absence of molecules. He also has found an experimental model using guinea pig hearts. He exposed the hearts to homeopathically dilute histamine, which affects the rate of blood flow.
>
> The fear aroused by Beneviste's work was verbalized in 1989 in a public forum. Philippe

Maliere, a scientist at France's prestigious Pasteur Institute said: "If these phenomena should enter our science books, it would, I fear, lead to an agonizing reassessment. I'm not ready to repudiate my work or science as we know it." Yet small breaks in the wall of orthodox medicine continue to appear. (The) February 9, 1991 article in the *British Medical Journal* presented the results of three years of research by three skeptical Dutch physicians. They did a world-wide search of all clinical studies on homeopathy and assessed them for the soundness of their methodology and results. They evaluated 107 controlled trials and decided that 16 of these were of high quality, with excellent controls. This included a 1986 study published in *Lancet*, which showed that mixed grass pollens diluted to 30C (to the 30th power) could have statistically positive results in the treatment of hayfever.

Most of the studies they had reviewed were done in the last ten years. The reviewers acknowledged that some positive results in some of the studies were acceptable, but they concluded, "if only the mechanism of action were more plausible." This leaves homeopathy as a treatment approach that often works, but no one can fully explain why it does so.

Homeopathy is a regular part of the training of present-day Naturopathic physicians, whom I shall describe in the next chapter. Two young (West) German M. D.s two years ago told me that their national health insurance pays for homeopathic treatment. There are many books and training guides for both laypersons and health practitioners available in the United States through the Homeopathic Educational Services in Berkeley, California. The National Center for Homeopathy in Washington, D. C. offers training programs for health professionals. The American Institute of Homeopathy is an organization of medical doctors and dentists who specialize in homeopathy. The American Medical Association does not consider homeopathy an acceptable method of treatment, however, because it is not based on present-day scientific principles.

Two years ago I undertook a homeopathic evaluation with a naturopathic physician in a nearby city. I was curious to see the procedure for myself. I did not have any medical problem at the time.

The one condition I thought might be helped or modified was a chronically stuffy nose, probably due to an anatomical problem, a deviated nasal septum, which I have had since adolescence. This resulted, in retrospect, to be an unreasonable application of homeopathy, since it makes no claim to cure a structural problem. Nonetheless the experience was worthwhile and informative. I underwent an extensive and thorough history-taking in my homeopathic evaluation, longer than is usual in conventional medicine. All aspects of my health were reviewed. After more than an hour of being questioned, I was informed that the doctor would study my responses and arrange a brief revisit in a few days. On the second visit I was given a small bottle of a homeopathic remedy made from a highly dilute amount of a natural element that had been manufactured according to standard homeopathic methods of dilution and succussion, and according to the United States Homeopathic Pharmacopeia.

Succussion is the term that refers to the tapping or striking of the solution in a container before it is again diluted several times, to reach a specified strength. Homeopathic practitioners traditionally believed that succussion transformed the potential energy of the substance into kinetic energy. Dilution and succussion are thought to release the kinetic energy of a substance. This theory might explain why no molecules need be present to have an effect.

There are several homeopathic pharmaceutical companies that produce homeopathic remedies. Since the substances are all extremely dilute by conventional standards, they are usually harmless as chemicals. They can, therefore, be sold or purchased without a regular prescription. They are regulated by the Food and Drug Administration in the United States. There are a few homeopathic substances that are illegal in the United States, such as Homeopathic Cocaine and Cannabis, even when extremely dilute. There are some homeopathic preparations that are no longer sold as over-the-counter substances.

Poisons such as strychnine and arsenic can be made into homeopathic medicines, and are entirely harmless, since the dilution of the original amount is so great that there is no risk. This is why the Bushmaster snake venom can be used as a medication.'Whether these and other homeopathic remedies produce positive results is a more complex issue. Responses can vary greatly from individual to individual. This depends on the skill of the homeopathic practitioner, who matches the remedy to the particular individual. Ten patients with apparently identical problems might each be prescribed or advised to take a different homeopathic remedy. This would depend not only on all the physical factors of the patient, but also on their individual mental and emotional symptoms or personality characteristics. In this respect homeopathy is a holistic system.

Dr. Kristy Fassler, a naturopathic physician, has given me an example of the criteria for evaluation of homeopathic remedy response. Homeopathic medicine is used frequently as a part of her practice, as is true for many naturopathic physicians. She states:

> The homeopathic practitioner has clear guidelines for assessing the response of the patient to a medicine. This evaluative procedure is part of what is known as Hering's Law of Cure. According to this set of observations, in a true healing process symptoms follow these patterns:
> (1) From above, down the body (i.e., from the head to the extremities),
> (2) From within to without (often in the form of discharges and other eliminative proc esses),
> (3) From the most important organs (i.e., the heart) to the least important organs (such as the skin),
> (4) In reverse order to their appearance, the chronologically most recent being replaced by those of the earlier stages of the disease, and commonly, earlier in the patient's life.
>
> Thus, for example, a patient healing from asthma, may develop sinusitis or eczema. This is healing from within to without and from the more important organ, the lung, to the less important organs, sinuses or skin. This would be seen as a curative response to treatment. Conversely, if a patient with eczema develops asthma, the patient is experiencing suppression rather than a curative response, because the body's symptoms are being driven deeper into the organism.

Andrew Weil, M. D. describes his own experience as a patient of homeopathic treatment in the first chapter of *Health and Healing* (Weil, 1988). He devotes the next two chapters to further discussion about homeopathy. He acknowledges the problem of determining why it works, even when it works. He also examines many other healing systems besides homeopathy. He suggests there are several principles that all therapeutic systems have in common. Belief in treatment is a significant factor that runs through all the elements of healing systems, though it is not the only factor.

The recent advances in the biochemistry of the nervous system and the immune system support the role of the mind/body connection as important in both the causation of disease and its cure or improvement. Yet, homeopathy does not require belief in it for effectiveness. Infants, toddlers, and animals have experienced its curative effects without any intellectual knowledge about it.

Dr. Kristy Fassler informed me of a veterinarian who had been successful in treating animals with homeopathic medicine. I met a woman recently who raises Sheltie collies. She spoke in positive terms about the value of homeopathic remedies prescribed by her veterinarian for her dogs.

The final word on homeopathy is still far along into the future. It is appealing increasingly to many people, and to some health practitioners. Some American M. D.s have studied homeopathy and have incorporated it into their practices, despite its unscientific status. A few years ago several M. D.s had their licenses suspended because of their use of homeopathy. This is becoming somewhat less of a threat for conventional physicians in recent years. As mentioned in Chapter 2 the state of Alaska has passed a law that permits M. D.s to use methods that are not proven scientifically, so long as they do no harm. Such use is not to be considered as unprofessional conduct. Charges of unprofessional conduct can lead to the loss of, or suspension of, a license to practice medicine.

Bach Flower Remedies and Flower Essences: Edward Bach, M. D. was a British physician who developed an unusual and distinctive form of homeopathy, known as the *Bach Flower Remedies*. Few homeopathic practitioners include it in their practice, since it is used more for emotional and mental problems than physical ones. Dr. Bach used it for patients with physical problems as well, and obtained good results. Over a period of about eight years of intensive research from 1928 to 1935 he developed thirty-eight homeopathic remedies derived from the flowers of several plants, bushes and trees.

Dr. Bach had first distinguished himself as a highly successful bacteriologist and practitioner in London over a period of twenty years. He had developed the successful use of vaccines against intestinal bacterial infection. In 1919 he accepted the position of pathologist and bacteriologist at the London Homeopathic Hospital, where he remained for three years. During these three years he discovered the writings of Hahnemann and was deeply moved by them, and felt a strong resonance with the concepts. Bach became increasingly committed to homeopathic practice and research. Hahnemann's emphasis on treating the patient and not the disease rang true for Bach.

Dr. Bach developed homeopathic remedies, called *nosodes,* derived from bacteria. He was so successful in his private practice that some colleagues called him "the second

Hahnemann." He continually conducted research to improve his effectiveness. He came to believe very strongly that temperament and personality were major factors in the development of physical illnesses.

He was a deeply spiritual man who believed that nature or God would provide the answers or substances for maintaining health or alleviating illnesses. He wished to find natural substances to replace the bacterial preparations he had been using. He also had a strong intuitive side to his personality and abilities. By 1928 he had found the first three plant substances to replace his bacterial remedies.

At first he created homeopathic forms of remedies from seeds, but later he was able to discover intuitively that freshly obtained flower blossoms were more satisfactory. He gave up his practice in London in 1930 and moved to Wales. It was there that he developed his method of using flowers. He gradually found other flowers to include in his treatment program both in England and Wales (Weeks, 1979).

Bach tried out different flowers by collecting the dew on the flowers before the sun had time to evaporate it. He experimented on himself with different flower remedies. Eventually, he found it equally effective to take fresh flowers, place them in spring water in a bowl, and expose them to the sun outdoors for about four hours. The water would then be placed in small bottles with equal parts of brandy. This would be the concentrated form, from which a few drops could be diluted in water to make a therapeutic solution. The dilutions were not as large as had been used in traditional homeopathy nor were the remedies following the Law of Similars as defined by Hahnemann. The Law of Similars required that large amounts of the remedy would produce symptoms similar to the illness for which they were to be prescribed. After Bach had discovered the first nineteen flower remedies, prepared with the use of sunlight, he then discovered the next nineteen. These were prepared by placing the flowers in boiling water and simmering for an hour.

The unique feature of Bach's flower remedies was their use to correct specific emotional or mental attitudes. Dr. Bach was convinced that early correction of mental or emotional attitudes or states would prevent the development of physical illnesses. A corollary was that distressed mental states eventually will manifest as physical illness. These mental states included lack of confidence, remorse, fear, terror, and many others (Weeks, 1979).

The first seven major mental categories, as defined by Dr. Bach, and some matching homeopathic flower remedies were as follows:

1. Fear: Rock Rose and Mimulus
2. Uncertainty: Cerato and Scleranthus
3. Insufficient interest in present
   circumstances: Clematis
4. Loneliness: Water violet and Impatiens
5. For those oversensitive to influence
   and ideas: Agrimony and Centaury
6. Despondency and despair: Larch, Pine, Elm and Willow
7. Over-care for welfare of others: Chicory and Vervain

Edward Bach, as described by those who knew him personally, was a deeply compassionate human being as well as a physician and researcher. Nora Weeks, who was one of his assistants, has written a fascinating small book about him, *The Medical Discoveries of Edward Bach, Physician* (Weeks, 1979).

The ideas and practice of flower remedies have been enlarged by the addition of American flower essences, developed by Richard Katz in Northern California in the 1970s. Katz, a student of spiritual traditions and humanistic psychology, created seventy-two flower essences and founded the Flower Essence Society.

Bach's flower remedies are listed as over-the-counter remedies in the Homeopathic Pharmacopeia. Rescue Remedy is the best-known. It is popular both in England and in the United States. It is composed of five flower essences. It can be used for any acute shock or upset by taking five drops under the tongue at frequent intervals following a trauma, either physical or mental, or an injury. As with other homeopathic remedies there are few scientific studies that prove the validity of these substances, in contrast to pharmaceutical drugs. Flower essences can be used along with any other medical or surgical treatments.

As modern science progresses in its understanding of mind/body unity, with more research in psychoneuroimmunology (PNI), Dr. Edward Bach's intuitive contributions may some day be more acceptable and even "make sense." Meanwhile, some citizens find homeopathy and flower remedies a useful adjunct to their program of health maintenance and treatment for chronic physical and emotional problems.

6

Naturopathy

The source for many principles of Western medical philosophy is usually credited to Hippocrates. He lived in Greece in 400 B. C. The Hippocratic writings consist of many volumes that bear his name. Other writers may have written some of the books besides Hippocrates. He was the first physician in the Western tradition to suggest that supernatural forces were not the cause of illnesses. He proposed more down-to-earth reasons, including the environment and internal bodily conditions. The ancient Greek gods were previously blamed for epilepsy or convulsive seizures. Hippocrates declared that it was due to natural causes, even if he didn't understand the process.

He emphasized the use of natural methods in the treatment of illnesses, such as proper nutrition, rest and exercise. He also declared that Nature is the source of healing. He and his disciples called it "Vis medicatrix naturae," the healing power of Nature. This included the actions of healing mechanisms in the body and mind that could maintain and restore health. This viewpoint is one source for the development of naturopathic medicine. The same principle is present in the Eastern healing systems of China, Japan, and India, as later chapters will elaborate. This viewpoint occurs in many other cultures throughout the world that are non-industrial, including most of the Native American (Indian) tribes.

The ancient Egyptians, Greeks and Romans used herbal remedies, therapeutic diets, water cures (hydrotherapy), exercise and many other natural techniques. Modern forms of naturopathic medicine are a blend of folk wisdom, ancient wisdom, and modern science. Naturopathic physicians do not prescribe pharmaceutical drugs, in the modern sense of the word. Therefore one can call such treatments drugless. Naturopathic physicians usually do no surgery. They do employ modern laboratory tests and X-rays.

The term, *naturopathy*, was coined by a nineteenth century German homeopath, John H. Scheel. He believed that the word implied health promotion and treatment of the whole person by natural means. Scheel came to the United States and helped in the establishing of naturopathy as a distinct and separate profession in 1900. A group of followers of Father Sebastian Kneipp also supported the development of naturopathy in the United States. Kneipp had been successful in Germany in developing a system of hydrotherapy, or water-cure in the 1890s.

Besides a variety of hydrotherapy methods, Kneipp's system included treatments using light, fresh air, and herbal teas. He also urged his patients to walk barefoot on wet grass, and run on snow, followed by a brisk massage to increase circulation. The Kneipp practitioners in the United States decided to widen the range of methods to include all natural methods of healing that could be used.

John Scheel had opened the Sanitarium Badekur in New York in 1895. In 1896 another German, Benedict Lust, who had been sent to America by Father Kneipp, opened the Kneipp Water-cure Institute in New York City. Lust had lived in Woershofen, Germany. He had contracted tuberculosis, undertook the Kneipp water-cure, with hot and cold packs, and recovered.

In 1898 Lust graduated as an osteopath from Universal Osteopathic College. By 1902 he founded the American School of Osteopathy, and ran a school of chiropractic and a school of massage in New York City. His enthusiasms also included creation of a magazine, *The Naturopath and Herald of Health* in 1902. In it he wrote:

> "Naturopathy" is a hybrid word. It is purposely so. No single tongue could distinguish a system whose origin, scope and purpose is universal—broad as the world, deep as love, high as heaven. . . we plead for the renouncing of poisons from the coffee, white flour, glucose, lard, and like venom of the American table to patent medicines, tobacco, liquor, and the other inevitable recourse of perverted appetite.

In 1914 Lust also received the M. D. degree from the Eclectic Medical College of New York. In 1919 Lust founded the American Naturopathic Association. The ideas and practices of naturopaths maintained some popularity until about 1937, when specific pharmaceuticals such as the sulfa drugs were introduced for infections, as well as anti-biotics in 1944. The specificity of potent pharmaceuticals for acute infections obscured the value of naturopathy. It is less effective for crisis conditions and of greater value for chronic conditions or for conditions not otherwise treated rapidly by conventional medicine.

Life-style management and proper eating habits were less dramatic in their effects on health and illness than the new "wonder drugs." With the support of the American Medical Association, court decisions were made severely limiting naturopathy. Yet there was and still is in Germany today, a well-established health-care practice of about five thousand practitioners derived from the nature cure movement. These practitioners are called "Heilpraktiker" or health practitioners. There are naturopaths also in many other countries including England, France, and Australia.

Until the mid-1950s naturopathy was frequently associated with chiropractic. Some chiropractors took an additional year of training and became certified as both naturopathic physicians and chiropractors. This trend ended in the 1950s. There had been ten naturopathic schools in 1950, some of which gave correspondence course degrees. This contributed to tarnishing the overall reputation of naturopathy. By 1960 all but one school had closed. In 1956 the National College of Naturopathic Medicine opened as an accredited school. After some years of struggle and several relocations it finally established a permanent home in Portland, Oregon. It was for awhile the only accredited school with a four-year graduate program and accepted for licensure.

In 1968 the National Association of Naturopathic Physicians estimated there were three thousand to five thousand naturopaths in the United States. The National Association dissolved in 1979, and the present national organization, the American Association of Naturopathic Physicians was founded in 1986. The total number of members is small but is growing steadily each year. A second fully accredited college of naturopathic medicine, John Bastyr College, opened in 1978 in Seattle, Washington.

It is the first new four-year naturopathic college in more than twenty years. The curriculum for the first two years of both schools is similar to conventional medical schools in many subjects. In the third and fourth years, however, the training is different. Students study herbal medicine, nutrition, homeopathy, natural childbirth, naturopathic manipulative techniques, and some electives in Chinese medicine, including acupuncture. There is also training in psychological counseling, more than in conventional medical schools.

There are limits to naturopathic health care, since it does not include trauma surgery nor other major surgery. Life-threatening infections would usually not be treated by a naturopathic physician, but mild and chronic infections can respond to naturopathic treatment. Most naturopathic physicians are primary care physicians. They treat both acute and chronic illnesses and also teach patients health maintenance techniques and principles. Some naturopathic physicians have received certification in midwifery.

Since the late 1960s naturopathy has had a gradual but steady rebirth with more legal and social acceptance. This is particularly true as the holistic health movement has grown along with a slow ground-swell of dissatisfaction with conventional medicine. Other forces in American society have also been an impetus to the growth of naturopathy. The ecology movement, the Women's movement and the publication of *Our Bodies, Ourselve*s also were supporting factors. The small size of this profession does not diminish the important role it plays as a direct challenge to the prevailing culture, both medically and in general. The training of a naturopathic physician is the only one for professional health-care physicians that includes extensive focus on clinical nutrition as a basic part of their training. That the naturopathic physician has chosen to spend seven years of education geared toward a career in natural medicine deserves attention. It is the only professional training that encompasses a training in holistic medicine. At present there is no such entity for study within conventional medicine.

Eight states and the District of Columbia now have specific licensing laws for the practice of naturopathic medicine. Montana has just recently approved a licensing law for naturopathic physicians. Oregon, Washington, Alaska, Hawaii, Florida, Montana, Arkansas, Connecticut, and the District of Columbia have licensing laws. Licensing proposals have been made for some other states.

The scope of naturopathic medicine was outlined by Bill Tribe in his article on naturopathic medicine in *The Holistic Health Handbook* (Tribe, 1978). He lists four broad categories that are not intended to be a complete list of natural therapeutics:

Physical
>   Hygiene
>   Ail methods of physiotherapy, including heat and cold, light, water, ultrasound and electricity
>   Manipulation of joints and soft tissues
>   Massage
>   Therapeutic and remedial exercises
>   Minor surgery

Neurological
>   Spinal manipulation
>   Acupuncture and acupressure
>   Reflexology and pain control

Psychological
>   Counseling
>   Hypnotherapy
>   Biofeedback and autogenic training

Biochemical
>   Corrective nutirition, including dietary supplements
>   Vitamins, minerals, enzymes, glandular extracts, and hormones
>   Botanical medicines
>   Homeopathic therapies

"Building health cures disease" is a common expression in naturopathic literature. Emphasis is placed on the maintenance of health or prevention of disease through education of the patient in nutrition, mental hygiene, physical fitness, and other aspects of bodily care. As Joseph Boucher, N. D. states in *Naturopathic Medicine: A Separate And Distinct Healing Profession* (Boucher, 1978): "Naturopathic medicine is very much in favor of all modern, scientific advancement and techniques (many of which verify naturopathic concepts and principles in use for hundreds of years) that extend the life and health of the human body, provided such scientific endeavors do not violate natural or biological principles."

Dr. Boucher further states, "The naturopathic physicians of modern times do not discard a method simply because it is old; neither do they immediately embrace a technique because it is new, popular, and heavily advertised. The methods of naturopathic medicine have been rigidly tested upon the anvil of time and experience." This supports the continued use of herbal or botanical substances that have been known for centuries in different parts of the world.

There are at least six major principles of Naturopathic Medicine. I have already mentioned Hippocrates "healing power of Nature." Another principle is also derived from Hippocratic teachings: Do no harm. This not only refers to avoiding harmful treatment methods, but also for present-day naturopathic physicians, adequate referral to other health-care professionals when indicated. Since the naturopathic physician does not prescribe pharmaceuticals with potent side-effects, there is less risk of iatrogenic (doctor-caused) illnesses.

The principle of "do no harm" is not limited to naturopaths, since I had learned this principle while in medical school. Unfortunately, as much as allopathic or conventional physicians wish to practice the same principle, it is not always possible or easy to prevent harm, due to the high incidence of damaging side-effects that may occur either from highly technical and complex surgical procedures or with the use of potent drugs.

A third principle is to find the cause as well as a diagnosis of the disease itself. Cause may relate to diet, life-style or habits of the patient. The goal is to identify and remove the underlying cause of an illness, not only to eliminate or suppress the symptoms.

A fourth principle is that of holism, treatment of the whole person. This includes attending to emotional, environmental, dietary and life-style factors, and physical factors. The fifth principle has already been mentioned, prevention of illness. This leads to the last principle, the doctor as teacher. The word, doctor, literally means "teacher." Educating the patient, with emphasis on self-responsibility, is a common practice in naturopathic medicine. This is also a basic part of any other type of holistic medical approach.

The modern growth of naturopathic medicine is reflected in the increasing number of states who license naturopathic physicians. The annual convention of the American Association of Naturopathic Physicians and the publication of a journal, now in its second year, are further expressions of this growth. It is understandable that naturopathic medicine struggles at times against the cultural climate that has emphasized a scientific world view that demands proof.

The naturopathic colleges and the naturopathic profession have had a significant impact on the natural foods industry and product manufacturers. This has occurred both through encouraging research and participation in research for and by natural foods industry and product manufacturers. This has helped to end false claims and establish appropriate ones more clearly. There is also bridge-building occurring between conventional medical centers and naturopathic training centers. Research on AIDS is occurring at the University of Washington Health Sciences program and John Bastyr College. The naturopathic profession itself is embracing a new research paradigm through the establishment of in-office protocols for single-disease management studies of consecutive cases.

In Australia there are naturopaths who practice herbal medicine and other natural therapies. Compared to Great Britain and the United States, the role of natural therapists is stronger in Australia, according to A. Hunter, N. D., a lecturer in herbal pharmacology in the Southern School of Natural Therapies in Fitzroy, Australia.

There have been studies on the safety, effectiveness and cost effectiveness of naturopathic methods. One evidence for the safety factor is the incidence of malpractice suits, which are extremely rare against naturopathic physicians in recent years. Some of this is understandable since surgery is not performed nor are pharmaceutical drugs prescribed. Referrals to other physicians have been appropriate and timely so that this has not been a cause for malpractice suits being filed. Cost effectiveness studies of three common diseases: middle ear infection in children, rheumatoid arthritis, and hypertension, have shown no greater expense. Frequently a somewhat lower cost is present for treatment and medications than conventional medicine.

Naturopathic medicine has established several specialties, each with its own society:

1. The Homeopathic Academy of Homeopathic Physicians (HAHP)
2. American College of Naturopathic Obstetricians (ACNO)
3. Naturopathic Physicians Acupuncture Association (NPAA)

The coming decades are likely to see more appreciation and acceptance of naturopathic medicine and its practitioners, as more citizens look for ways to maintain their health, and seek less costly approaches to the treatment of illness. There will, of course, continue to be a need for surgical interventions and specialized medical treatment from conventional M.D.s when indicated.

7

Herbal Medicine

"Have you tried cayenne?" was the cook's suggestion to J., a woman who was attending a workshop at a conference center in Maine eleven years ago.

"What? Did you say 'cayenne'?" This was not a discussion on preparing a Mexican recipe. The food at this conference center was vegetarian, a part of the center's emphasis on health enhancement. Besides being an excellent cook, the young woman was also knowledgeable and interested in herbs for healing.

J., the guest, had been scheduled for a hysterectomy in a few days. She had been troubled by heavy and constant uterine bleeding due to fibroids, a common non-cancerous tumor of the uterus. J. had thought she was adequately prepared for the several days of the conference, but discovered she had miscalculated the amount of "sanitary supplies" she needed. Also, she had agreed to participate in a lengthy and intensive workshop, called The Enlightenment Intensive, which lasted fifteen hours a day for three days. No one was to leave for any reason while it was meeting. Even car keys had to be turned in to the office. Therefore, she asked the cook if she or other staff, were going to town to shop. If so, would they pick up some additional sanitary pads for J. She gave the cook a brief explanation of the problem she was having and thus the question, "Have you tried cayenne?"

The cook explained that cayenne could possibly solve the problem. She explained how to swallow four teaspoons a day of cayenne pepper, also known as red pepper.

"Begin with one quarter of a teaspoon swished around in water and swallowed quickly without breathing, followed by some more water. Next dose increase to half a teaspoon and so on up to one teaspoon four times a day. If it is going to work, you will know in forty-eight hours."

J. proceeded to do this. By the time she left the conference two days later she was almost free of any bleeding. The next day at home there was no bleeding at all. She called the surgeon and the hospital to cancel the operation that had already been scheduled for two days later.

About five years later there was a mild return of symptoms. Again J. took cayenne pepper for several days and again she became free of abnormal bleeding. I know this account is accurate since J. is my wife. As she says, "I still have all my parts and pieces."

This is by no means a suitable treatment program for all women with fibroids. Anyone considering such an approach needs to have complete information about their medical condition, and have had a thorough medical examination and workup by a gynecologist, before undertaking a less conventional approach. Nonetheless it does show the possible use of an herb or plant for medical treatment.

The use of cayenne by the American Indians was common. They used it for arrow wounds and other external lacerations, as well as consuming it for internal use. Putting cayenne in one's socks in the winter will keep the feet warm! I first learned about the difference between black and red pepper when one of my daughters came home from college in California. She had taken a course in health and self-care. The instructor included some discussion of herbs and had talked about cayenne. It surprised me to hear that cayenne is gentler on the stomach than black pepper, despite the sharper taste of red pepper. All peppers are not the same.

Most of us are familiar with a few herbs from reading recipes in newspapers and magazines. Fewer people are familiar with the use of herbs for treating illnesses. References by elderly grandmothers or greatgrandmothers may recall the use of some herbs for the relief of common ailments.

The more detailed use and value of medicinal herbs is far less commonly appreciated. There are worldwide trends, however, that reflect a revival of knowledge and use of herbs for healing. Before the turn of the century, and even into the twentieth century, the use of plant substances was a significant part of conventional physicians' treatments. As an increasing number of drugs were isolated from plants, and eventually synthesized, and as antibiotics were synthesized, physicians considered herbal remedies too nonspecific and not standardized sufficiently to be of value. Few conventional M.D.s today know much about herbs for healing. Naturopathic physicians, however, use them frequently.

By contrast there are an increasing number of citizens who are studying the use of herbs through correspondence courses or study at schools of nonconventional medicine such as colleges of Oriental Medicine. In a city near my home there is a store that sells over two hundred commonly used herbs for anyone who wishes to use them for health maintenance or for relief of symptoms. The owner is a trained herbalist who can recommend or inform the customer what the traditional teachings are about any particular herb or combination of herbs. Some acupuncturists are graduates of schools of Oriental medicine. During the three-year program they also study Chinese herbal medicine.

Conventional physicians throughout Europe two or three hundred years ago were critical of women healers who used herbal remedies extensively. This was during a time when there were no women physicians. The male physicians who had been educated at university schools of medicine were the most vocal in their disdain for the women herbalists.

One English physician in 1775 agreed to accompany his fiancée to a woman herbalist's shop. Here he learned that the foxglove plant was especially useful for people suffering from Dropsy. This was a term for anyone with swollen feet and ankles. The foxglove plant is rich in digitalis, still a useful drug for congestive heart failure. The physician was William Withering. He is credited in the annals of medical history for the discovery of digitalis in 1775 for the treatment of heart failure and heart disease. His fiancée and the woman herbalist did not get any direct credit. Until the 1920s digitalis leaf, obtained from the foxglove plant, was the only form available.

In the 1800s close to eighty percent of pharmaceuticals contained elements derived from green plants. Even today about twenty-five percent of pharmaceuticals is so derived. If antibiotics from molds are included, the percentage rises to forty-one percent. In Germany and other European countries, and in Japan today, physicians use herbal and plant substances more than in the United States. In France at the University of Paris Nord there is a chair or department of herbalism. Several large companies in France and Japan produce herbal preparations. Silybum marianum, milk thistle, is a commonly prescribed plant for liver ailments. For hearing disorders gingko biloba is prescribed. It is also used for circulatory problems that affect the brain and contribute to dementia. Gingko increases blood flow to the brain. Scientific journals have reported these effects, besides those mentioned by herbalists.

Herbal medicine is not a substitute for conventional medicine by any means. Nonetheless, there are many herbal preparations that are useful for the relief of bodily symptoms if used with proper knowledge, or competent advice is obtained. In the United States herbalists are not licensed as a separate professional practice. Besides independent herbalists, there are health food stores and herbal shops that sell herbs and may give advice. The quality of the advice ranges from questionable to highly knowledgeable.

Herbalism is an example of naturopathy, since herbs often function as a means to stimulate the body to return to balanced health, and aid natural healing. Often no specifically defined illness is treated but only the symptoms experienced by a person. Even for the same illness a highly individualized approach may be taken. This is similar to homeopathic treatment, which focuses on the person who has the illness more than the disease by itself.

In the Hippocratic writings at least two hundred and fifty medical plants and their uses are described. Later a Greek physician in the army of the Emperor Nero of Rome wrote a book on herbs in which he listed six hundred plants. Galen, physician to the Emperor, Marcus Aurelius, in the second century A. D. was an outstanding herbalist whose methods were used for fifteen hundred years.

In today's scientific climate it is easy to dismiss herbs as only of historical interest but of no real value. This is clearly not true, but their use requires a different approach than is usual in crisis medicine where results are expected rapidly and predictably. Andrew Weil, M.D., author and practicing physician in Tucson, Arizona, lectures at the University of Arizona medical school on complementary and alternative healing systems. In his excellent, informative book, *Natural Health, Natural Medicine* (Weil, 1990), he describes his use of botanicals for prescriptions. He estimates that he has recommended or given out botanical substances forty times more often than a prescription for a pharmaceutical drug. He has not seen a single adverse reaction with distressing side-effects from herbs. He credits his accumulated knowledge as having come from herbalists, naturopaths, American Indians, and non-conventional healers. It is also a help that his undergraduate major was in botany, a subject rarely studied by pre-medical students.

There is a growing skepticism and caution by some citizens towards synthetic drugs, invasive surgery and technological diagnostic procedures. Yet there are few experts available to consult about curative herbs. As will be discussed in a later chapter, Traditional Chinese Medicine, Japanese Kampo medicine, and Ayurvedic medicine of India make active use of herbs in their treatment programs. Synthesized pharmaceuticals have a distinct advantage in being pure and highly potent, and also measurable. This is also what unfortunately contributes to the frequent occurrence of undesirable side-effects. These lead to iatrogenic (doctor-caused) diseases and death. The benefit/risk ratio is always a constant concern for physicians as well as for patients. Physicians usually inform their patients of at least some of the risks inherent in the use of either drugs, diagnostic procedures, or surgical treatment.

Every drug produces a desired effect as the primary goal. All other effects are defined as "side-effects." Unfortunately, these are direct negative effects, defined as "untoward side-effects." Although often only unpleasant, occasionally they are dangerous. I once characterized a new psychiatric drug as having a "minor side-effect, death." My facetiousness was meant to underscore the dangerous side-effect that the manufacturer clearly listed, a decrease in white blood cells, which could lead to death if unchecked. A close monitoring of the blood count by weekly checkups would detect this and the drug would have to be stopped. The manufacturer listed this in all its advertisements to physicians. The drug might be used for persons with severe forms of schizophrenia who had not responded to any of the other drugs available. This decrease in white cells, leukopenia, occurs in 1 out of 100 persons.

My intention is not to suggest that this particular medication should never be used, since it may be the only medication to which some individuals respond. Hearing the danger of this drug described as a side-effect makes it sound less ominous than it is. In the 1970s a senior research director of a pharrmaceutical company was quoted as saying (Lucas, 1974):

> We've come full circle. Back in the 1880s fully 80% of medicines were plant-derived. Gradually researchers turned more and more to chemicals, both organic and inorganic. Today half the curatives in the average medicine cabinet are products of somebody's test-tube, and only 30% are plant based. Now, almost out of desperation, we're going back to nature—back to plants. For good as the test-tube is, it hasn't cured man's greatest cripplers-arthritis, heart disease, severe mental illness, asthma and cancer.

In the fifteen years since that comment there has been progress in newer drugs for heart disease and cancer, but the statement is still valid. The "war on cancer" has not been won by any means nor have other crippling diseases been cured.

Large drug firms continue to research the tropical jungles for roots, leaves, barks, and seeds that might produce new cures for some ailments. A concern about the destruction of the Amazonian rain forest is the possible loss of plant species that have not yet been examined for possible medicinal value. In 1938 curare was discovered in the jungles of South America, where it had been used by some native tribes as a poison for centuries. It became a valuable drug in anesthesia as a muscle relaxant for several decades.

Scientific research is analytical, taking things apart and examining them in minute detail. Substances are isolated so that they can be purified and measured accurately to determine their effects in a predictable and controllable way. This becomes essential since the isolated substance is so much more potent than the whole plant from which it is derived.

Morphine is a natural substance in the Poppy plant, from which opium is also derived. It was first extracted and isolated in 1803 by a German chemist. It was declared the active ingredient, with twenty-one other inactive ingredients. Fifty years later, in 1853, Alexander Wood, M.D. of Scotland invented the hypodermic syringe. Unfortunately, his wife became the world's first morphine addict.

At least two other useful drugs are also present in opium and therefore are not inactive after all. One is codeine, a milder narcotic than morphine, and frequently prescribed by dentists after tooth extraction for pain relief. The other drug present in opium is papaverine, used to dilate blood vessels, and prescribed by heart specialists for persons with coronary artery spasm.

The use of an herb often requires much longer time for the desired effect to occur. The chemicals in the plant are less concentrated than in an isolated drug. This does not allow for use in crisis situations such as an acute heart attack. Digoxin, therefore, is more effective and more potent than digitalis leaf. For more extended and chronic use, however, there could be advantages to a plant used in its entirety, such as digitalis, derived from the foxglove plant, rather than a synthetic drug, such as digoxin.

Few doctors today prescribe digitalis, which is still an excellent heart medication to bolster the heart and prevent the development or recurrence of congestive heart failure: Instead digoxin is used. When digitalis had been in use, the first sign of overdosage was nausea or vomiting. Only in later stages of overdosage or poisoning did abnormal heart beats occur. Since digitalis has been replaced by digoxin, there is no early warning and no nausea occurs. Sometimes progress through chemistry can have some shortcomings.

Herbal preparations are more useful for chronic and mild conditions rather than acute medical problems. The benefits derived from a whole plant or herb are often greater than the value of each separate chemical substance contained within it that can be extracted separately. There is an interaction among the various substances that does not occur if each is separate. The use of crude preparations, when taken by mouth, also has the effect of releasing the active ingredients slowly into the bloodstream. The low concentration and the presence of inert compounds slow down absorption. This is the reason for less side-effects. The biochemical actions of a plant depend on all the organic and inorganic substances in it.

It is difficult sometimes for physicians to credit Nature with intrinsic wisdom. In so-called primitive cultures and in past centuries before the era of science, many people believed that the immediate environment could provide for them, including what they needed for reestablishing health when ill. In the 1700s a Methodist minister in England was inspired to seek the cure of "swamp fever" by looking for a cure near the swamps.

He noticed that the willow trees grew vigorously along the banks of the streams. This led him to try out the use of the bark of the willow. In doing so he obtained some definite results with certain cases of fever. The willow bark contains salicylic acid, which is close in chemical structure to aspirin, acetylsalicylic acid. This is not the usual approach to pharmaceutical research, but nontheless one cannot dismiss practical results altogether.

Modern-day diuretics are a common type of drug prescribed for high blood pressure, and to eliminate excess fluid in the body through increased urination. A common risk, or undesirable side-effect is the "washing-out" from the body of potassium, which can lead to potassium depletion, and in extreme form, cardiac arrest. The heart normally requires a proper amount of potassium to function. Prescribing extra potassium is often necessary with some diuretics. Nature, however, offers dandelions as a diuretic. The French word for dandelion is "pis-en-lit," or "pee-in-bed." As a child I recall being teased by another child that if I touched the dandelions, I would wet my bed! Folk truths are conveyed without anyone knowing where the knowledge comes from. Dandelions examined chemically contain three times the normal amount of potassium contained in most ordinary green-leaved plants.

The methods for preparing herbal medicines vary. Some terms are familiar, such as infusions and tinctures. There are others that are known only by herbalists or members of past generations. When you soak a tea-bag in hot water, you are making an infusion. Traditional herbal infusions are usually prepared by taking one or two ounces of dried herb in a pint of boiling water, and steeping for fifteen to twenty minutes. A cupful is then consumed three to four times a day. An example of herbs that are used for infusions are goldenseal, used for inflammation of the stomach and intestines. Marshmallow and comfrey can soothe irritation of the gastro-intestinal tract. Agrimony and shepherd's purse will soothe damaged tissue and stop diarrhea. Cowslip and lemon balm are used to reduce mental stress.

The tincture form of preparation is used for many modern herbal preparations. These are prepared with alcohol and water, so that ten drops of the tincture in a few ounces of water are equivalent to several cups of tea, or infusion. Although more expensive than dried herbs, the potency is better preserved, and a small bottle can last for a month's use.

A decoction is another form of preparation used for bitter substances or a mineral salt. This is produced by soaking the herb or substance in cold water for several hours, and then bringing to a boil, followed by simmering for half an hour. Honey may be added as a sweetener. Half a cup before meals is a common prescription.

Fomentation is the term for a hot pack. I learned and used an excellent hot-pack technique from a macrobiotic counselor, who advised the use of ginger compresses for a stiff neck. Freshly grated ginger is placed in a small cheese-cloth bag and then dropped into several quarts of boiling water for twenty minutes. Towels are then soaked in the gingered water, wrung out and placed on the body for fifteen to twenty minutes. Both the heat and the ginger in combination can give relief. The ginger apparently increases the blood flow and allows deeper penetration of the heat.

Anyone whose childhood was in the 1930s, and perhaps in the 1940s, may recall being given a mustard plaster on the chest for the relief of a bronchitis or "chest cold." The irritation of the skin stimulates the lungs and bronchi to open up more and give relief. It is unlikely that many pediatricians today would recommend it, since there are many medications now available that "do the same thing."

I might have preferred a mustard plaster a few years ago when I experienced a wheezing during a cold that was accompanied by some mild bronchial irritation. I have never had asthma, and was totally unfamiliar with the experience of wheezing. This was slightly alarming, so I consulted a family practitioner, who gave me a sample of medication, which contained Theophylline, a commonly used medication for lung problems of an asthmatic type. Although the sample suggested one tablet twice a day, he advised me to take two twice a day. I did experience a cessation of the wheezing, but the side-effect of jitteriness and anxiety-like feelings was more uncomfortable than the wheezing. I reduced the dosage but still felt very jittery. I decided to live with the wheezing for another day or two, without the benefits of the drug. Perhaps a mustard plaster would have been more comfortable.

Herbal preparations are made from different parts of the plant, depending on the particular species. A few examples of parts a herbs are:

1. Flowers: Chamomile,   comfrey,   marshmallow
2. Leaves: Dandelion,   comfrey,   marshmallow
3. Bulbs: Garlic
4. Roots: Echinacea,   wild yam
5. Fruit & Berry: Cayenne,   saw palmetto,   hawthorn

The proper use of herbs also may require some dietary changes as part of a larger program of treatment. Herbs appear to enhance the body's response to improved dietary habits. It is worth noting that not all herbs are entirely harmless. As with other medications high doses can be poisonous. Licorice is not only a candy but also is used as a healing herb. In large doses, however, it can be harmful to the liver. Comfrey is also dangerous if taken excessively. For most herbs this is not usually an important issue.

At times it is difficult to make a clear distinction between herbs and other plant substances, such as fruits, vegetables and other food supplements. Evening primrose oil and black currant oil are natural sources of a fatty acid, gamma-linolenic acid, not easily obtained in ordinary diets. They can be an aid to health or in the treatment of some illnesses. These oils are reported to help some individuals with arthritis, auto-immune diseases, and premenstrual syndrome. As with many herb preparations, it requires several weeks to as much as eight weeks to produce positive results.

Aromatherapy: The whole herb, or its extract, is the common form for use as part of a medical treatment. Less frequently known and used, the essential oils are substances derived from plants that can be used in herbal medicine. A separate field of study and application, aromatherapy, has developed with the use of these oils. It is both an ancient practice and a new one. The use of incense and aromatic oils has been known for centuries in India and ancient Egypt. The conscious planned use of aromas for healing is a more recent development in Europe and America. Most herbalists do not use essences, or essential oils. In England the National Institute of Medical Herbalists does not teach the use of essential oils. Essential oils are more familiar in their use as room fresheners, in the bath, and in massage, but also can be useful as home remedies for many minor ailments. Since France is the country where aromatherapy has developed more than in other countries, it is not surprising there are general practitioners in France who have trained in aromatherapy. The world center for the cultivation and extraction of essences is in southern France. The pioneer of aromatherapy was René-Maurice Gattefossé, a chemist, who explored not only the cosmetic uses of essences but also their antiseptic properties.

Gattefossé made a discovery by accident (Tisserand, 1977) when he was carrying out an experiment in his laboratory. An explosion burned his hand severely. He immediately immersed his burnt hand in pure lavender oil, and noted that the burn healed at a very fast rate without any infection and no scarring. He published his first book, *Aromatherapie* in 1928.

As described in Robert Tisserand's The *Art of Aromatherapy* (Tisserand, 1977), Gattefossé reported in 1938 the experiences of a colleague, who had set up an aromatherapy clinic in Los Angeles. Reports of cures of skin cancer, gangrene, and facial ulcers were described. Bites from Black Widow spiders could be rendered harmless due to the use of lavender oil. Tisserand reports that the lavender oil combines chemically with the spider venom to form a harmless compound. This also has been applied to snake and insect bites.

A French M.D., Jean Valnet, had already used herbs in his medical practice. He was inspired by Gattefossé's work also to use essences in his professional treatments. He had treated battle wounds in World War II with essences. It is through Dr. Valnet's efforts that aromatherapy has become more fully established. Dr. Valnet wrote a book in 1964, *Aromatherapie*, with the same title as Gattefossé's 1928 book. There also have been Italian researchers who have shown clinically the positive effects of essences in anxiety and depression.

Essential oils can be taken by mouth, used in massage, inhalations, and baths. Since so much of physical illness can be stress-related, the degree to which oils help people feel better and more relaxed also may contribute to better healing in general.

Essential oils are often anti-bacterial. They also may act similar to acupuncture in creating a better balance of energy throughout the body. This is more difficult to demonstrate scientifically. The concept of energy flow and energy balance is a more Eastern or Oriental viewpoint and not readily accepted by most scientists. This may change over the next several decades as Vibrational Medicine (Gerber, 1988) is more acceptable.

Well-known uses of essential oils include oil of cloves for toothache, peppermint oil for indigestion, and eucalyptus for inhalations to relieve nasal and bronchial congestion. External applications, however, are the most common forms of use.

Several aromatic gums, herbs, and their essential oils came into medical use during the eighteenth century. During the nineteenth century, however, new chemicals replaced many natural products, and the perfume industry had greater interest in the use of aromatic substances. With the more recent developments in aromatherapy, there is a return to medicinal uses of essential oils.

There are two kinds of effects produced by essential oils. One is physiological and the other is psychological. The physiological effect may be through the nervous system or by acting directly on an organ or tissue. Some oils stimulate salivary secretion, such as cloves, lavender, mint and rosemary. Some have anti-spasmodic and laxative effects. There are oils that have an effect on the heart and circulation, such as camphor, calamus and hyssop oil. Studies have been conducted that demonstrate the effects on the lymphatic system, endocrine system, urinary tract, and the nervous system.

The use of essences for relief of disturbed emotional states has been extensively developed. Tisserand lists some in his book (Tisserand, 1977):

Anxiety, nervous tension:	benzoin, bergamot, camomile, camphor, cypress, geranium
Depression, melancholy:	basil, geranium, jasmine, newroli, patchouli, rose
Confusion, indecision:	basil, cypress, peppermint
Fear, paranoia:	basil, clary, juniper, jasmine
Grief:	hyssop, marjoram, rose
Jealousy:	rose
Suspicion:	lavender

The combination of essential oils with massage can be enhancing to the value of the massage, both for physical and psychological reasons. It is understandable that oils have become a part of skin care and cosmetics more than medicinal treatment in the twentieth century. Good skin care, however, is more than attractiveness or esthetics, and does have a role to play in maintaining health, both physically and psychologically. Essential oils are effective in treating skin conditions because they are readily absorbed into the deepest layers. Bergamot, lavender and juniper can act as astringents and antiseptics for acne and severe oiliness of the skin and scalp. Some oils can be too irritating to the skin unless used in very dilute form, such as camphor or eucalyptus. Frequently essences are mixed with vegetable oils for proper use.

An article in the *New York Times* business section in September of 1991 described the expanding sales of essences by several corporations. One Japanese herbal and essence company has developed a computerized system for introducing various aromas into office buildings and hospitals for both psychological and physical purposes, through the air-conditioning and heating equipment. Homes can be subjected not only to room fresheners to decrease unpleasant odors, but have selected aromas distributed into rooms to enhance relaxation and calmness. This can contribute to health as well as pleasure.

The most popular aromas in a home have always been those wafting out from the kitchen when someone is preparing a meal of one's favorite foods. Even without any herbs or spices, many foods are tasty due to their aromas. Good food is both nourishing to the body and to the emotions, and even to the soul. The definition of which foods are nutritious, however, can sometimes be controversial. It used to be said that everything that is pleasurable is either "illegal, immoral or fattening." Nowadays we have to add "cancer-producing."

8

Nutrition

The consumption of food is neither illegal nor immoral. At times it can be fattening and there is now clear evidence that high-fat foods contribute to the development of some cancers, especially breast, colon and prostate cancer. This makes food more than a matter of necessity or pleasure, but intimately related to health and disease. Still, for many people it is not that tasty a subject, unless they are hungry. Nutrition sounds even less appealing unless one has scientific curiosity. The dictionary defines nutrition as "The process by which a living organism assimilates food and uses it for growth and for replacement of tissues."

Food is also big business in many ways. Tobacco companies have been buying up food manufacturing companies increasingly in the United States as less of the population smoke cigarettes. The meat, dairy and sugar industries have powerful lobbies in Washington, D.C.

As a teenager living in New York City, I often enjoyed dining at foreign restaurants. My favorites were Japanese, Indian, and Mexican. There were Chinese, French, other European, and Near Eastern restaurants available as well. In those days I never thought of food as having any connection to health, other than for obesity or starvation.

In high school biology I learned about the basics of food digestion, simple biochemical processes, and a little about vitamins and their function. In college chemistry and biology there were more details. Finally in medical school I studied biochemistry extensively. In one laboratory experiment we were given a dish of fresh uncooked scallops. We were asked to extract the glycogen from the scallops and measure the quantity. Glycogen is a chemical that is stored in the human liver as a pre-cursor of sugar, which can be quickly converted into glucose as the body needs it. Scallops have a high content of glycogen and therefore could be used to study the nature of glycogen and its conversion into sugar. I tolerated the sacrifice of a tasty seafood dish in the name of scientific learning. This was the most vivid linkage between food and medical education that I can recall. There were no separate courses in nutrition. While studying the treatment of some diseases, particularly metabolic diseases, such as diabetes and hepatitis (liver inflammation or infection), dietary requirements or modifications were explained. Otherwise there was little consideration of the role of diet and nutrition in the development of diseases and their treatment.

Today the time allotted to the study of nutrition in medical schools is not much different from several decades ago. Until recent decades there has been little scientific proof that diet had much of a role in the development of disease or its treatment, except a few obvious situations such as severe malnutrition, excessive obesity, and vitamin deficiencies. Nutrition has more often been associated with health issues and prevention rather than illness and disease. Medical training focuses on detecting and treating diseases and minimally on prevention.

Although brief lip-service is given to Hippocrates as the Father of Medicine, his actual ideas are not usually studied in medical school. Only in recent years did I learn that Hippocrates declared: "Let food be your medicine." In a 1990 article on unproven methods in the treatment of cancer in a publication of the American Cancer Society, high fat diet was stated as a contributing factor for cancer of the colon, breast and prostate. It also emphatically declared that this does not mean to suggest that diet has any specific role to play in the treatment of cancer. The article was on macrobiotic diets and its use by patients with cancer.

The belief that diet lacks direct value as a treatment approach in cancer and arthritis continues to be the prevailing view of most physicians. Demonstrating the benefit of diet as a specific element of treatment for cancer or arthritis is difficult. The methods used in scientific research favor the isolation of a single element rather than studying complex processes. Dietary research is a complex and difficult type of study, since there are so many variables. Despite this there are observational studies that lend support to the value of food and nutrition in the treatment of many diseases. There is also increasing evidence for the role of diet in the causation of disease.

The report in 1977 of the U. S. Senate Subcommittee on Nutrition, the McGovern Committee report, *Dietary Goals for the United States,* summarized many studies relating nutrition to health and illness. Although it was cautious in its recommendations for how Americans should eat, it did propose a number of changes in the content of the American diet.

Less fat, cholesterol, sugar, and salt were among its most important declarations. The dairy and meat industry spokespersons made critical rebuttals to these suggestions, somewhat similar to the tobacco industry's earlier rebuttals to the Surgeon General in 1964. At that time he had declared that smoking caused or contributed to the development of lung cancer. The Surgeon General in 1989, C. Everett Koop, M.D., produced the publication of the first *Surgeon General's Report on Nutrition and Health.*

The report's main conclusion is that overconsumption of certain dietary components is now a major health issue for Americans. The excessive consumption of fats was particularly of concern, at the expense of foods with complex carbohydrates and fiber, such as vegetables, fruit, and whole grain products. The report pointed out that dietary factors played a prominent role in at least five of the ten leading causes of death for Americans: heart diseases, cancers, strokes, diabetes mellitus, and atherosclerosis (hardening of the arteries). The report was particularly concerned with chronic diseases, which are steadily increasing in incidence every year. The report was developed for the use by policy makers more than individual citizens. Nonetheless every citizen would find benefit in knowing the contents of the report. The Summary and Recommendations section of the original 750-page report is available in a 171-page book, including recipes and menu plans (Warner Books, 1989).

The report acknowledges that the precise contribution of diet to the development of coronary heart disease, strokes, diabetes, some cancers, and atherosclerosis (hardening of the arteries) is uncertain, since there are multiple causes for many chronic diseases. Nonetheless there are compelling reasons for a need to change dietary habits. Three-fourths of deaths in the United States are due to chronic diseases. Death itself may not be enough of a threat for many people to make changes in their eating habits, or any other life-style activities. The risk of impairment and loss of comfortable living may stir some people to action. The Surgeon General's report is relatively conservative, since it relies only on acceptable scientific findings, and avoids the more anecdotal types of studies, which may be suggestive and sometimes useful, but not as convincing or reliable as scientific studies.

The three major conclusions of the report are:
1. Improvements in diet can reduce chronic disease risk.
2. Similar dietary recommendations apply to virtually all chronic diseases.
3. Reduction of fat intake is the first dietary priority.

The ability and willingness of people to use information that will improve their health and prevent disease is one of the most challenging problems. Not only making dietary changes but also other life-style changes is involved. Many individuals can say what is nutritionally good for them. Yet detailed questioning of what people actually eat often contradicts their declared knowledge.

The sources of saturated fat in the diet consist of meat, which accounts for 35 percent of the total saturated fat, dairy products 20 percent, and cooking and table fats and oils 34 percent. To follow the recommendations of the Surgeon General's report would require leaner meats, poultry and fish, dairy products with lower fat percentages, and increased intake of fruits, vegetables and grains. Despite some changes, such as skim milk and less beef consumption, the average amount of saturated fat eaten has not decreased. It has remained the same over the past fifty years. More cheese and more ice cream replace some of the other changes. At least half of all Americans eat red meat on any given day, and more than 40 percent eat high-fat lunch meats. With the increase in salad dressings and table spreads the actual fat consumption has been increasing.

Fruits, vegetables and grains are far from popular with most Americans. Early childhood experiences have a strong influence on eating habits. This includes negative conditioning from poorly cooked or overcooked vegetables, parental pressures to "eat your spinach," and cultural habits. Studies show that forty percent of Americans eat no fruit on a given day. Almost fifty percent eat no vegetables other than potatoes, beans, or salad. Eighty percent do not eat any high-fiber bread or cereal. Some people have responded to questionnaires by including ketchup as a vegetable! Ketchup is about fifty percent sugar in composition. Since the government agencies define what ketchup is, any health-food store ketchup that contains no sugar must be labelled as "artificial ketchup."

Despite these somewhat dreary statistics, more of the public are becoming health-conscious about food. Food is a multi-billion dollar industry. The health-food and natural food industry are small compared to the major food manufacturers. Nonetheless, like leaven in bread, citizen awareness is growing slowly. Large fast-food chains such as Wendy's have introduced salad bars, and MacDonald's has invested millions into developing leaner hamburgers. These are not massive breakthroughs but they can contribute to consciousness-raising for some people.

When salt and sugar are abundantly supplied in baby foods, the infants and children develop strong preferences for food with these ingredients, despite what is ultimately healthy. Commercial baby foods until recently were high in salt and sugar, sometimes to satisfy the parent's taste more than the child's. The kinds of food the infant and child are fed at home obviously condition them as well. There are other strong influences as well that affect all members of a family, such as advertising, and the actual processing of foods. A scanning of many labels in supermarkets will reveal how frequently processed foods contain salt, sugar, and many other ingredients that were not present when the original food was grown or raised as meat, vegetable, or cereal. The estimated number of chemical additives present in processed foods is about two thousand.

The five major recommendations of the Surgeon General's report of 1989 are:

1. Fats and cholesterol: Reduce consumption of fat (especially saturated fat) and cholesterol. Choose foods relatively low in these, such as vegetables, fruits, whole grain foods, fish, poultry, lean meats, and low-fat dairy products. Use food preparation methods that add little to no fat.

2. Energy and weight control: Achieve and maintain a desirable body weight. To do so, choose a dietary pattern in calory intake which is consistent with expenditure of energy. To reduce intake, limit consumption of foods relatively high in calories, fats, and sugars, and minimize alcohol consumption. Increase energy expenditure through regular and sustained physical activity.

3. Complex carbohydrates and fiber: Increase consumption of whole grain foods and cereal products, vegetables including dried beans and peas, and fruits.

4. Sodium: Reduce intake of sodium by choosing foods relatively low in sodium and limiting the amount of salt added in food preparation and at the table.

5. Alcohol: To reduce the risk for chronic disease, take alcohol only in moderation (no more than two drinks a day) if at all. Avoid drinking any alcohol before or while driving, operating machinery, taking medications, or engaging in any other activity requiring judgment. Avoid drinking alcohol while pregnant.

The recommendations are basic and conservative. They focus on long-term prevention and do not consider other health considerations directly such as "high-level wellness." There also can be less disabling symptoms that may be distressing, such as food allergies and sensitivities, gastro-intestinal disturbances, mood disturbances related to diet, and other less life-threatening health problems.

There are some Americans, and many citizens of other parts of the world, who face the problem of undernutrition, if not actual starvation. For most Americans the more likely problem is overeating, and unbalanced eating. Besides the influence of eating patterns on leading causes of death, there is the never-ending social, medical and nutritional problem of alcoholism. There are three additional causes of death associated with excessive alcohol consumption. Alcohol can cause death because of cirrhosis of the liver, accidents, and suicide. In 1987, of the 2.1 million deaths in the U.S., nearly 1.5 million were due to the five diet-related conditions and the three alcohol-related ones.

Recent nutritional knowledge suggests that many Americans consume more protein than is necessary for good health. The recommended amounts by the National Research Council are 44 grams for women and 56 grams for men. These figures are difficult to translate into actual food amounts but can be used for comparison at least. The average intake in the United States per day is 60 grams for women and 90 for men, obviously more than desirable. There is evidence that excessive protein intake contributes to calcium loss from the body. This is a major cause of osteoporosis, a problem for women over fifty, and for men over seventy.

High intake of fat is not only a contributing factor in some cancers constantly on the increase, such as breast cancer, cancer of the colon and cancer of the prostate, but also a factor in obesity and gallbladder disease. When I was a medical student, I worked one summer in a small hospital in Arizona on the Navaho Indian reservation. The most common disease that was diagnosed at the hospital was gallbladder disease, cholecystitis. For most of these it was a surgical problem because of gallstones formed in the gall-bladder, a small pouch or bag under the liver. The gallstones were mostly formed from cholesterol. What was remarkable was the frequent occurrence in slim young men besides the more familiar cases of middle-aged women who were overweight and had several children.

The impact of "civilization" on the Navaho led to their buying much of their food supplies at a local trading-post. There they purchased white flour, sugar, and oils. Much of their cooking consisted of fried bread and fried mutton, with a liberal use of refined white sugar and coffee. The limited supplies of water also may have contributed to some dehydration, which might have also aggravated their overworked gall-bladder.

All the scientific truths that have been discovered in recent years about food are of little value unless people can apply them. This demands attention to more personal and human factors, which involve taste, flavor and the style and quality of cooking. Cookbooks are constantly among the most popular of books that are printed and sold. A major problem in reducing fat in a person's eating habits is that much of tastiness and good flavor often comes from the fat in the food.

In September of 1991 the *New York Times* reported in the business section about "The Long Hard Quest for Foods that Fool the Palate." As the writer of the article, Eben Shapiro, stated: "The expression, 'Having your cake and eating it too,' has become an urgent battle cry for the food industry." He describes the food industry's search for fat substitutes, such as MacDonald's use of leaner beef mixed with carageenan, derived from seaweed. Other substances derived from beef are also added as flavor-enhancers.

The fat-substitute industry may grow to more than a billion dollars in several years, it is reported. A race is on between several manufacturers to produce leaner beef and pork products that will still please the palate of the consumer, and also be healthier. Attempts to produce a satisfactory ice cream or frozen dessert with less fat and fewer calories has been a struggle. Taste comes ahead of any other consideration for most of the public. The movement of the food industry toward being a technology industry led one investment expert to call food "software for the microwave."

Americans' consumption of fat today makes up about forty to fifty percent of their calories. The recommendations of the American Heart Association and the American Cancer Society are for a limit of thirty percent, a cautious figure. There are individual experts among both the medical profession and other nutritional spokespersons who recommend twenty percent. Nathan Pritikin, who developed the Pritikin Diet for people with coronary heart disease, recommended as low as ten percent. This approaches an almost dangerous level because the body has a definite need for some fat and cholesterol to manufacture cell walls, and maintain several other physiological processes of the body.

Cookbooks alone cannot help a person make a transition to a healthier and life-preserving style of eating. There is a need for both self-education through reading books and pamphlets, attendance at lectures and workshops in cooking and food preparation, and intelligent presentations of recommendations found in the books. The psychological aspects of food are a major force in shaping what we choose to eat, or what we eat unconsciously without any thought.

The increasing diagnosis and incidence of eating disorders in the United States is a worrisome phenomenon. There are no conclusive explanations for the increase. The richness of the American diet may often make it difficult for many people to maintain a healthy and appropriate weight, and therefore increase the preoccupation with obesity for some. Anorexia nervosa is a term for a condition that literally means "nervous lack of appetite." The persons who suffer from this condition, usually young women fifteen to thirty-five years of age, do not have a lack of appetite, but rather have a profound wish not to eat, usually for fear they will become fat-looking. The preoccupation sometimes approaches a delusion and at other times it is more of an anxiety and fear. Anorexia nervosa is diagnosed if a person loses twenty-five percent of body weight or is twenty-five percent below the average for their height, accompanied by the fear of looking overweight. There are profound physiological changes in the body as a result, including loss of menstruation. There can be a ten to fifteen percent death rate among such patients. It can occur occasionally in young men.

Another type of eating disorder is bulimia, in which the person, most often a young woman, binges on food, and then purposefully gags herself and throws up what she has eaten. In bulimia there are similar fears of gaining too much weight. These two conditions are not common or normal types of nutritional disturbance, but they may reflect some of society's attitudes toward obesity and appearance. Psychologists and psychiatrists mainly deal with these problems, and only secondarily by nutritionists.

Sugar intake is a major factor in producing a large percent of dental problems throughout the world. The problem of adequate dental care to prevent loss of teeth over a long period of time is important. Diet clearly plays a part in prevention. Because of costs and lack of dental insurance, many people seek little to no dental care during their lifetime, unless they develop acute problems. These are often the result of long term neglect. As a consultant to a nursing-home with an elderly population, I find it obvious how troublesome it can be for many elderly to have to deal with dentures instead of their own teeth. This affects not only the kinds of food they can eat, but also their appetite and their general ability to consume food. Many elderly who live by themselves may be in even greater distress, and develop nutritional deficiencies, since they cook for themselves and do not always get a balanced diet. The old expression, "For want of a nail, the shoe was lost; for want of a shoe the horse was lost; for want of the horse, the country was lost," can apply to dental care, nutrition and health.

The Surgeon General's Report and the earlier Senate Subcommittee report make no reference or suggestion that citizens should consider becoming vegetarians. It might appear almost un-American. The word itself frequently suggests a strange cult-like quality, especially when it is presented as "vegetarianism." It has been associated with religious groups throughout the world at times, and some famous people in history, such as Charles Darwin, Ralph Waldo Emerson, Albert Schweitzer, and George Bernard Shaw. Some modern-day show business people, authors, sports heroes, and musicians have also been vegetarian. None of this has much meaning to the public in general and rarely inspires many to change their patterns of eating.

Despite the caution and conservatism of the medical profession and other professional organizations, there are some physicians and an increasing number of non-medical nutritionists who are declaring the usefulness of a predominantly, if not exclusively, vegetarian style of eating. A better description would be a diet of complex carbohydrates, with low-fat and less protein. This focuses on the quality and type of food-stuff. To eat a low-fat diet and less protein than the usual American diet, it becomes necessary to eliminate almost all meat, including poultry and fish, and eat more vegetables, beans, and grains. A reduction in refined sugar and small amounts of alcohol are also part of this type of diet.

Initially this sounds austere to most people and is not an approach that can be undertaken overnight. It flies in the face of most of society's habits, and also the billions of dollars spent by the dairy, meat, sugar, and other food industries to advertise and sell their rich products. To make a clear and full case for the advantages of a mostly vegetarian diet would require more discussion than is possible here. I would like to describe briefly some books that present a highly convincing explanation for this viewpoint. In the coming years there will be many more books documenting and explaining how not only to live longer, but have more enjoyment in life through better health and more energy. These words may sound in themselves like a sales pitch but the knowledge that has been accumulating about diet and disease is massive. As a well-trained nutritionist, Ranan Cohen, recently told me, "There is enough nutritional research at present to last for ten years, without any more being done."

A highly readable author on nutrition is John McDougall, M. D. of St. Helena, California. I have heard him speak, both at a lecture and on his eight 1988 audiotapes on "The Truth About Good Health and A Miracle Cure For Disease." Dr. McDougall's first book, *The McDougall Plan* (McDougall, 1983) presents very clearly, with extensive scientific references, the case for a vegetarian diet. He is stricter than most of the medical profession today. His ideas are compelling and are particularly valuable for anyone who has already developed signs of any of the many "degenerative" diseases that are so common today, including diabetes, heart disease, and cancer. He expresses more concern with prevention and teaching a health-supporting type of diet. His second book, *McDougall's Medicine, A Challenging Second Opinion* (McDougall, 1985) focuses more directly on the use of diet in seven major disease conditions.

In describing how he came to his convictions about proper diet for health and the alleviation of many illnesses, he states in his lectures that it was not due to his personal experience as much as his clinical work as a general practitioner on a Hawaiian planta-tion for three years. He did experience a stroke at eighteen, which he related to his excessive weight and extremely rich diet. He eventually overcame most of the effects of the stroke. This did lead to a change in diet. What reinforced his thinking and made explicit the role of diet in illness were his observations of three or four generations of plantation workers in Hawaii. Most of the most elderly workers were born in Japan, China, and the Philippines. Their children and grandchildren, and sometimes even greatgrandchildren, were born in Hawaii. Dr. McDougall noticed that the oldest genera-tion was the healthiest. The younger the generation, the more diseases were present. The life-styles were not strikingly different in the younger generations but the diet was clearly different.

The oldest generation ate mostly rice and vegetables, with little to no meat, fats, or refined sugar. The younger ones increasingly ate the mainstream American-style diet. As far back as 1944, one of the few treatments for high blood pressure that had some effect, before there were any medications, was Dr. Walter Kempner's rice diet. He noticed how much less high blood pressure occurred among traditional Oriental popula-tions at the time, and inferred that it was related to the large amount of rice in the diet, and the absence of meat. For Americans then and now, eating only rice and some grape-fruit was not an easy diet to follow, nor was it a very complete diet. Dr. Kempner, how-ever, could get positive results, and has continued to treat patients over the following forty-five years at the Kempner Clinic in Durham, North Carolina. In Jane Heimlich's 1990 book, *What Your Doctor Won't Tell You* (Heimlich, 1990), she reported that Dr. Kempner at 85 was still directing the program.

There have been studies of Japanese living in Tokyo, Hawaii, and Los Angeles. The incidence of high blood pressure, and cancer of the colon and breast, have increased in these populations as they have moved west. Changes in diet were obvious. It is also a possibility that life-style and stress were also involved.

Unlike some types of strictly controlled scientific experiments, it is rarely possible to declare that diet alone or stress alone is the cause of a disease, such as high blood pres-sure or cancer. The commonly used term to describe this is "multi-factorial." Nonethe-less Dr. McDougall and others make a strong case for the value of changing dietary habits for the prevention of disease. There is also a place for nutrition in the treatment or alleviation of many diseases.

The average person faces a problem with the many books available that advise so many contradictory directions about nutrition. The greatest confusion exists in the large number of "Diet" books on the market that promise to help people lose weight. There is a marked distinction between dieting books and the ideas and facts presented by Dr. McDougall. Anyone who shifts their eating habits to include more grains and complex carbohydrates, with significant reduction in fats and sugar, can eat as much as they wish in order not to feel hungry. They will still lose excess weight, and have a reduction in cholesterol, if it is higher than normal. There are no "secrets" for improving health or obtaining a proper weight. All the facts necessary are readily available. The problem, as always, is being able to apply them.

Dean Ornish, M. D. is a cardiologist who has presented impressive scientific findings to support the value of a more vegetarian-type diet. The conclusions of his extensive research of fourteen years present a slightly more liberal diet than Dr. McDougall, but still support everything that I have found in Dr. McDougall's writings. Dr. Ornish has conducted the first scientific research that demonstrates a method to reverse heart disease, without surgery or drugs. His 1990 book, *Dr. Dean Ornish's Program for Reversing Heart Disease*, reports in detail the program he carried out with a group of patients with proven blockage of their coronary arteries. He also includes specific diets and an extensive recipe collection for following his recommendations. His program was not only a very low-fat, vegetarian diet, but also included stress reduction, exercise, and support group meetings for the patients. Some Yoga exercises and meditation were also part of the program.

I heard Dr. Ornish present his findings in 1988 at the annual meeting of the Society for Behavioral Medicine in Boston. The only casualty in his research program was a man who drove himself so fiercely that he pushed himself on a rowing machine vigorously for an hour and died an hour later. He also had the most difficulty of all the patients in sharing feelings in group discussion. He had followed the diet and exercise components of the life-style program. Some of this program was shown to the public on the Nova series of the Public Broadcasting System in the Fall of 1991.

Neither the title nor the subject of the book does justice to Dr. Ornish's presentation. He deals extensively with the emotional aspects of heart disease in a profound and sensitive manner. His program is called "Opening Your Heart." This touches on the emotional and spiritual aspects of heart disease, its prevention and treatment, as much as the details of proper diet, exercise, and group support. Issues of intimacy and sharing are as important as right diet and right exercise.

What Dr. Ornish could prove with the patients that went through his Opening the Heart program was measurable reopening of the blocked coronary arteries. This was accompanied by clinical improvement in most of the patients. When he first applied for research funds for the program from several research foundations, he was told that it would not be possible to reverse heart disease, and even if it could be done, one year is not long enough to prove it. Life-style changes may reduce the risk of getting heart disease, it had been previously believed, but not to reverse it. This is exactly what he did prove could be done.

The control group, who did not participate in the program, was asked to follow their doctors' advice: to make moderate dietary changes, to exercise moderately, and to quit smoking. After one year, repeat angiograms were made, showing the degree of blockage of the arteries. A large number of the experimental group who made the comprehensive life-style changes showed some reversal of their coronary artery blockages. In contrast, the majority of the control group, following their doctors' advice, became measurably worse a year later.

One of the oldest participants, a seventy-four year old man, had greater improvement than many younger ones. Among the younger participants, one with severe blockage showed marked improvement, as good or better than many others.

There are many other fascinating and important findings reported by Dr. Ornish. His dietary principles and practices are striking. The percent of fat in this program's diet was very low, usually ten percent, as he reported in a lecture that he gave to the Society for Behavioral Medicine in 1988. An entire chapter is devoted to the diets used in the research. After two further chapters on how to quit smoking and how to exercise, the remainder of the book consists of a cookbook, with careful instructions on how to move gradually into the type of eating presented by the many recipes.

The Reversal Diet is the one used by the participants in Dr. Ornish's research program. The Prevention Diet is for those who want to keep from getting coronary heart disease. The diet is also useful for decreasing risks of several other common diseases. Besides preventing or decreasing the risk of such diseases, there is also a more positive aspect. Both diets are capable of improving the quality of life in a positive manner. Most people following them tend to eat fewer calories than the average American. The Reversal Diet consists mostly of complex carbohydrates, or starches, along with grains, beans, vegetables and fruits. Most dietitians and alert laypersons are aware that fat adds weight more readily than sugar. Despite the constant advertising of the meat industry, there is no advantage to animal or meat protein over vegetable protein. Many outstanding athletes who are vegetarian have shown equal or even superior stamina and strength to their meat-eating competitors. Several years ago a Japanese baseball team in Japan was at the bottom of their league. When they got a new coach who switched the entire team to a grain-based and vegetable diet, they ended up the season in first place. In 1988 the American Dietetic Association issued a statement about vegetarian diets that stated:

> A considerable body of scientific data suggests positive relationships between vegetarian lifestyles and risk reduction for several chronic degenerative diseases and conditions, such as obesity, coronary artery disease, hypertension, diabetes mellitus, colon, cancer, and others . . . Vegetarians also have a lower rate of osteoporosis, lung cancer, breast cancer, kidney stones, gallstones, and diverticular disease.
>
> Although vegetarian diets usually meet or exceed requirements for protein, they typically provide less protein than nonvegetarian diets. This lower intake may be beneficial, however, and may be associated with a lower risk of osteoporosis in vegetarians and improved kidney function in individuals with prior kidney damage. Further, a lower protein intake generally translates into a lower fat diet, with its inherent advantages, since foods high in protein are frequently also high in fat.
>
> It is the position of the American Dietetic Association that vegetarian diets are healthful and nutritionally adequate when appropriately planned.

The control group of patients in Dr. Ornish's research was on a 30 percent fat diet and their condition worsened in a year. Dr. Ornish's research findings support Nathan

Pritikin's recommendation for a ten percent fat intake for the treatment of heart disease. The danger might be in someone following this strict a diet without proper medical supervision and not including the other components of Dr. Ornish's program. There is always a greater risk in following only one element of a program, whether for health maintenance or to decrease a disease process. Nonetheless, it remains true that a marked reduction in fat will improve health and heart disease.

The story of Nathan Pritikin's terminal illness is a dramatic confirmation of his ideas. Pritikin had much earlier in life developed severe coronary heart disease. This led him to the development of the Pritikin diet, which improved his health markedly, so that he lived for several decades after his original diagnosis. In the last few years of his life he developed leukemia, which eventually was the cause of his death. At the time of his approaching death, he did not wish to have any publicity resulting from his admission to a hospital. He therefore used a false name when he entered a university medical center hospital on the East Coast. He died during this admission. An autopsy was done without the pathologist knowing the deceased patient's identity. It was not customary to make a detailed examination of the heart in every autopsy, if the cause of death was not due to heart disease. Nonetheless there was a practice in this hospital to do a very thorough examination of the heart at certain intervals, such as every twentieth or hundredth autopsy. This was done and the results showed there was no evidence of any coronary heart disease in Nathan Pritikin's heart.

William Castelli, M. D., the director of the Framingham Heart Study, which began more than forty years ago and is continuing, reports that no one with a cholesterol less than 150 ever had a heart attack in the study. This level can be achieved on a low-fat vegetarian diet.

When calory intake can be reduced indirectly through changes in the makeup of one's diet, without dieting in the customary sense of trying actively to reduce calories, other benefits may occur. There is a lowered risk of cancer. Another possible benefit has been proposed by Roy Walford, M. D. Dr. Walford is Professor of Pathology at the University of California in Los Angeles. He has been particularly interested in gerontology, the science of aging research. His first book, *Maximum Life Span* (Walford, 1983) discussed the possibilities of extending the life span of humans. This is different from life expectancy, about seventy-five to eighty years in the United States for the white population. Maximum life span refers to the theoretical limit of human longevity, which is about 110, with rare exceptions. Dr. Walford in his second book, *The 120 Year Diet,* provocatively suggests that life span could be stretched to one hundred and twenty years. His goal is not so much to achieve this as to improve the quality of life lived to eighty or ninety. His program is one of calorie reduction at a very slow rate, taking four to six years to reach this. It is not designed to be an immediate reducing or weight-loss diet. Dr. Walford's views are not accepted throughout the medical profession. To lower calorie intake so there is a ten to twenty percent reduction in daily calorie intake for the rest of a person's life is a major task that most people would not relish undertaking. There is, however, a connection to what Dr. Ornish has proposed, since he noted in his program using the Reversal Diet that the patients tended to eat fewer total calories.

Dr. Walford has observed that animal experiments that fed mice on less than the usual calories led to an extension of life span by as much as fifty percent. It also fore-stalled many signs of aging in the animals. It has not yet been proven that this applies to humans. Dr. Walford himself has been following his own proposals of eating a lower calorie diet than usual. He defines the set-point of a person's weight as the prevailing weight that has been present for several years or decades. A person could very slowly reduce their calorie intake over four to six years so that the body weight gradually decreases and a person adjusts to a ten to twenty percent reduction in calories. The goal is a healthier quality of life in old age.

Gerontologists and geriatric physicians are declaring increasingly that old age is not inevitably accompanied by illness. Further, much of our images and ideas about old age are from images of impaired or ill elderly, and not old age itself.

In view of the rapidly increasing percent of the population that is over sixty-five and eighty-five (the fastest-growing group in the United States), good health would contribute to a greater degree of pleasure and comfort in the later years of life. It might still be a problem for those who reach the age of 114. A woman in England a few years ago was the oldest person known to the *Guinness Book of Records*. She was quoted as saying: "I don't know why the Lord is punishing me by having me live this long." She died shortly afterward and the record was passed on to a woman in the United States. She has not yet been quoted.

Information about nutrition outside the scientific and medical field exists that may be well worth exploring and studying. At times it can appear somewhat overwhelming and highly contradictory. While caution and some degree of skepticism may be necessary, it is not a reason to avoid them altogether. For example, a competent nutritionist informed me that Adelle Davis' books contain some excellent ideas about nutiriton and food, but I am not yet familiar with them. Frances Moore Lappe's *Diet for a Small Planet* was a revolutionary book in 1971. She did write a tenth anniversary revision in 1981, which decreased her original emphasis on food-combining. Nonetheless she made some important statements about the consumption of plant foods in preference to meats.

A more recent writer and teacher of "natural food" cooking and eating whose ideas I can recommend, and are consistent with most of the medical authors I have already described, is Annemarie Colbin. She has written a highly readable book for the average person interested in health and good eating, *Food and Healing* (Colbin,1986). She consulted several physicians in the preparation of her book. She also was influenced by the macrobiotic teachings of its founder, George Ohsawa, and his best-known disciples, Michio Kushi and Herman Aihara. She presents a useful description and critique of several diets, including the Standard American Diet (S. A. D.), the Pritikin diet, high-protein diets, the fortified natural-foods diet, and the macrobiotic diet. She presents in an understandable manner some concepts of Eastern (Oriental) diets. She also presents a primer on the use of food for healing several common conditions, as well as some general principles for healing. It is not meant to replace the use of physicians but can be very useful for some less serious conditions, and as adjuncts in the treatment of serious medical problems. She also discusses what are the effects of different foods on mood, sexuality, and the effects of food preparation. Her book is a contribution to raising awareness about food, often not given any consideration in our everyday hurried culture, with fast-foods becoming faster and degenerative diseases appearing in younger and younger members of the population. Annemarie Colbin has also written a companion book, *The Book of Whole Meals* (Colbin, 1983), which is a cookbook of natural foods, encouraging the exploration into not-so-fast and healthier foods.

In the United States many citizens know the largest ice cream company in the country, Baskin and Robbins. The founder's son, John Robbins, has written and lectured extensively throughout the United States about food and health in a way that challenges his family's business products. He was initially the black sheep in his family. In a talk he gave in 1990 at the annual summer conference of the Kushi Foundation, a conference centered on macrobiotic living, John Robbins described his journey as an exploration of how America eats, and the methods of production for the meat and poultry industry. He has also read a large section of the scientific literature that echoes what Dr. McDougall and Dr. Ornish are saying and writing. In addition, John Robbins writes with great passion about the horrors of the modern animal factories where cattle, pigs and chickens are processed. Reading his book might create a few converts to a vegetarian type of diet through negative conditioning. He also shows clearly what the medical literature is stating. It is a different reading journey than the more usual calm, objective presentations, but well worth the trip. He spells out in some detail the interweaving of politics, big business, and nutrition. There is a strong ecological element to his presentation that is not found in many medical or health writings.

There continue to be, and will be for a long time, many controversies within the medical profession about the role of nutrition and diet for health and the healing of illnesses. Naturopathic physicians are highly committed to the role of nutrition in maintaining health and the use of food as medicine. As we shall see in a later chapter this is especially true in the traditions of China and India. There are some physicians within conventional medicine who practice nutritional medicine. There is an entire subfield called orthomolecular medicine and orthomolecular psychiatry that uses doses, frequently in large amounts, of vitamins and minerals to treat a wide range of illnesses. The principles and practices of orthomolecular medicine are not accepted by most physicians, but nonetheless there are those who actively practice orthomolecular medicine, with some encouraging results. Some scientific studies do not support the claims. Some counterarguments by orthomolecular physicians are that the critics have not understood the techniques nor the findings, and so the debate continues. In chapter 2 I briefly described the experience of Rickie, the daughter of psychiatrist, Frederic Flach, M. D. She was significantly helped and ultimately cured with orthomolecular medicine and behavioral optometry.

The physician who was the founder and director of the Princeton Bio Center, Carl C. Pfeiffer, M. D., where Rickie was examined and treated, has written an extensive survey of orthomolecular medicine for physicians, *Mental and Elemental Nutrients* (Pfeiffer, 1975). I do not necessarily agree with all that I have read in his book, but it is a challenging presentation of how food and nutrients can affect many bodily and mental functions. There are presently several professional organizations of orthomolecular medicine.

It has been said that a specialist knows more and more about less and less. The field of medicine continues to be characterized by greater and greater specialization, except for a small trend by some physicians who have become family practitioners, which itself has been defined as a specialty. With specialization the medical profession has tended to leave nutrition to those who have specialized in it and have become established as registered dieticians. This is most clearly seen in hospital practice, since registered dieticians or nutritionists are on the staff of most hospitals. There are also registered dieticians in private practice throughout the United States.

For several reasons, including professional standards and a concern to protect the public, many states have passed legislation to limit the practice of nutritional advice to registered dieticians. This has led to controversy about who may speak about nutrition to the public. There are many who have not pursued formal education leading to certification as registered dieticians, and yet are knowledgeable about nutrition and diet. There obviously are others who can claim expertise but do not have it. As in all matters of advice-seeking and information-gathering, it is necessary to use common sense and caution. A health-food owner or clerk may be highly knowledgeable and intelligent, or may not be endowed with such qualities. Certification and licensing do offer certain minimum guarantees of expertness. The problem arises, as in many areas associated with holistic health and medicine, that scientific studies may not yet support ideas and practices that have been found useful and health-enhancing, but not yet proven. It may not be possible to know for sure whether an unproven method will eventually become acceptable and adopted by the medical profession, or will be shown to be useless or dangerous.

There are experts on nutrition who teach and write without traditional education in nutrition. Nathan Pritikin, an engineer, is one example of a person without formal nutritional training. His ideas have been helpful to many individuals with heart disease, before medical research established the correctness of his recommendations. Another person whose observations and practices are controversial, and not yet acceptable within conventional medical circles, is Dr. William Kelley, a Texas dentist. He developed a dietary treatment for cancer twenty years ago. A more recent exponent of Dr. Kelley's treatment method is Nicholas Gonzalez, M. D. of New York. Dr. Gonzalez is a well-trained physician, a graduate of Cornell University school of medicine, and trained in clinical immunology. Dr. Gonzalez spent six years investigating the records of ten thousand patients who undertook Dr. Kelley's dietary program for cancer. Dr. Gonzalez was sufficiently convinced of the usefulness of the Kelley diet that he conducts a practice in New York City based on Dr. Kelley's findings and recommendations. The diet is vegetarian-based, and includes extensive use of digestive enzymes. I do not have sufficient knowledge of it, however, to recommend it. Nonetheless it remains an example of a dietary approach to the treatment of cancer, totally unacceptable to present-day oncologists.

The macrobiotic diet has become increasingly well-known as another major nonconventional dietary approach to the treatment of cancer. It is also for the relief or treatment of many other chronic illnesses. Beyond its application for treatment it is also being used for health maintenance for adults and children. In its broadest application it has philosophical and spiritual elements that broaden its scope to a "Way of Life." The best-known and most published leader of the "Macrobiotic Movement" is Michio Kushi of Becket and Brookline, Massachusetts. Less well-known but also a teacher and writer of macrobiotics is Herman Aihara of Oroville, California. Both Michio Kushi and Herman Aihara were students and supporters of the founder of macrobiotics, George Ohsawa. Ohsawa grew up in Japan before World War II, spent part of his adult life in France and the United States, and lectured throughout the world. He was the author of three hundred books, some of which have been translated into English and French. He died in 1965.

Michio Kushi has had an influence beyond the specific field of macrobiotics. He was originally trained in International Law, and was deeply interested, as he still is, in world peace. He came to the United States in 1949. After living in New York for several years, he moved to the Boston area, where he founded the first natural foods company, Erewhon, which he later sold. He also started the *East West Journal,* which is still an active magazine devoted to natural food, health and living. Over the years he has established the Kushi Foundation and the Kushi Institute, which trains students to be macrobiotic counselors, macrobiotic cooks, and Shiatsu massage therapists.

Macrobiotics is today far from what its reputation had been in 1971 when it temporarily was given notoriety due to several individuals dying from a mistaken application of George Ohsawa's "Zen Macrobiotic" diet, which led to starvation. The developments by Michio Kushi, Herman Aihara and their hundreds of certified students in no way resembles Ohsawa's earlier advice, which apparently had not been correctly followed, or lacked guidance. Some textbooks of clinical nutrition today still refer to macrobiotics as a dangerous diet based on the two or three 1971 disasters. I have read many books by Kushi, Aihara, and others, attended four of the annual six-day summer conferences sponsored by the Kushi Foundation, and listened to many lectures by a wide range of macrobiotic experts. I have also sat at the mealtime table and chatted with over a hundred individuals who have followed the macrobiotic approach to eating and nutrition. I do not find any reason to think that there is any danger resembling the old stories to which I have referred. Sometimes too rigid an approach can be dangerous. I have met many individuals who were living with very advanced forms of cancer but were obviously thriving. Some reported that their physicians had often given them a very poor prognosis or expected outcome. There were also individuals who had suffered from serious intestinal illnesses, allergies, and arthritis. They reported remarkable improvements with their adoption of a macrobiotic diet.

I am fully aware, and need to point out, that these are not scientifically studied groups, and I do not have any statistics. For most of the forty years that macrobiotics has been developing, there have not been formal scientific studies. There now are several clinical studies of macrobiotics being conducted in several places in the United States. There are books by several individuals who overcame life-threatening and advanced cancers. These are detailed anecdotal reports that still are inspiring and worthy of attention. Anthony Sattilaro's *Recalled by Life* (Sattilaro, 1982), has been the best-known and perhaps the most remarkable, since Dr. Sattilaro described his profound skepticism about what he undertook. His professional medical training was according to biomedical and strictly scientific traditions.

His situation, however, was so desperate that he agreed to explore the use of a macrobiotic diet for his own illness. He was suffering from a very advanced stage of prostatic cancer, with spread to his skull and other bones of the body. He was only forty-seven when he was diagnosed with metastatic cancer. He wrote about his situation in detail and the subsequent course of action he took. Although he finally succumbed to the disease in 1989, he had lived eleven years from the time of diagnosis, which had previously been unheard of in view of the severity of his condition. He had obtained an extended remission with no signs or symptoms of his cancer for ten years. The cancer recurred only after he had abandoned the macrobiotic diet that he had been on while in remission, according to him. He then made an attempt to obtain another remission by returning to a strict healing version of the macrobiotic diet, but he could not repeat his first results.

I heard him speak in 1988 at the annual macrobiotic conference. Although he was obviously not well, he was remarkable in his energy, passion, and excitement about the journey he had been on over the past ten years. Others have reported his constant struggle between his viewpoints as a medically trained scientist and the totally different philosophy that macrobiotics expresses, and from which it is derived, namely, Eastern Taoist and other spiritual principles, also Eastern views of the body, mind, and spirit. He shares with the reader of his book his constant struggle, which he could never completely resolve.

The macrobiotic diet should not be a rigidly prescribed one, and in many respects resembles much of what Dr. John McDougall and others have proposed. It does include the use of sea vegetables and an active use of miso, a fermented soybean product. Some critics say that the diet is "too Japanese" for many Americans. While this is somewhat-true, there have been many adaptations in the use of the basic recommendations. These usually are a diet that is about 50 percent grains, 25 percent vegetables, 10 percent beans, and the rest includes miso, sea vegetables, some condiments, and a small amount of fish, but no dairy, meat or poultry, sugar, caffeine-containing beverages, and some limitations or avoidance of vegetables of the nightshade family, such as potatoes, tomatoes, eggplant, peppers and zucchini.

The macrobiotic approach demands commitment and study. Although there are many books available, it is advisable for anyone who might consider adopting it to attend lectures or obtain advice from a competent macrobiotic counselor. There are at least eight or more centers throughout the United States that offer counseling and lectures. There are also centers throughout many countries of the world. It has become an international movement. The use of macrobiotics for AIDS patients has been reported and there is ongoing research now established in several medical centers.

I have described my personal exploration of a year on a macrobiotic diet in an essay that I wrote in 1987. It was published with essays by nine other M. D. physicians in *Doctors Look at Macrobiotics* (Japan Publications, 1988). An introduction by Michio

Kushi gives an excellent summary of the macrobiotic philosophy and the specifics of the diet. Although I am not as close a follower of the diet as I had been, I do find the ideas and recipes a useful contribution to my eating habits and attitude. I have deep appreciation for what I have learned and gained from my exposure to it.

An excellent way to learn about and appreciate the breadth and scope of macrobiotics as both a diet and a way of life is to attend the six-day summer conference regularly sponsored by the Kushi Institute in Western Massachusetts. There is also an active program in California, including a summer conference, sponsored by the Vega Study Center, directed by Herman Aihara. He has also established and directs the George Ohsawa Macrobiotic Foundation in Oroville, California. They also publish a bimonthly journal, *Macrobiotics Today*. Ohsawa and his leading disciples, Kushi and Aihara, make a large contribution to the meeting of East and West in many respects. My brief comments do not do adequate justice to their abilities and writings. The value of macrobiotics in the rehabilitation of prisoners and criminals has been described in *Crime and Diet* by Michio Kushi (Kushi, 1987) and his associates.

Macrobiotics has been briefly described in this chapter on nutrition. It is most often referred to as a special kind of diet or nutritional viewpoint. It does, however, extend to a broader range of subjects related to health and healing, and to a spiritual viewpoint. Associates and students of Kushi have also written about massage, such as shiatsu or acupressure massage (Yamamoto, 1979); palm-healing (Kushi & Oredson, 1988), and human behavior (Tara 1985).

The teachings of Ohsawa and his followers do cover a truly holistic approach to living. Many Americans and Europeans are continually being drawn to explore and follow these teachings in order to find a larger or greater life, which is what the word, macrobiotics, literally means. A Western scientist understandably rejects most of what is presented, not only because of the absence of familiar scientific studies, but also the Western scientist cannot measure the "Chi" of traditional Chinese medicine, Japanese "Ki," nor the "Prana" of Indian medicine and philosophy. In the Eastern traditions these concepts of energy have been used for thousands of years, but not readily accepted at all in the West by biomedical scientists. Since the "reopening" of China during Richard Nixon's presidency there has been a much greater awareness of some of Traditional Chinese Medicine than previously. In China itself, even with modern Western medicine also fully accepted, there has been a revival of the much older non-Western healing traditions.

II

Eastern Traditions of Healing

9

Traditional Chinese Medicine

A famous early meeting of East and West was by Marco Polo who journeyed to China in the early 1400s. Europe and the Islamic Near East knew of China before Columbus. He struggled in 1492 to find Japan and the Far East by sailing west without success. He met native Americans whom he called "Indians," but he never reached the East. In the 1500s the Portuguese were frequent visitors to Japan until it was closed to Europeans for three hundred years. Admiral Perry of the United States Navy reopened the meeting of East and West in 1858 when he established diplomatic relations with Japan.

China had remained more open to the West during the centuries that Japan was not in active communication with European countries. This sometimes was to the detriment of China. The history of the interaction of the East and the West is charged with many complex cultural, economic, and political issues from the time of Marco Polo to the present. Shortly after World War II F.S.C. Northrop, professor of philosophy at Yale University, wrote *The Meeting of East and West*. He examined the cultures and countries of both the East, Near East, and the Western hemisphere. He tried to predict the trends of the coming decades of the post-war era. The subtitle of Professor Northrop's book was "An Inquiry Concerning World Understanding." Part of his concern was the issue of U. S.–Soviet relations in 1946 and their future. This was before the Cold War, the independence of India, and the establishing of Israel. Professor Northop saw both India and a future Israel, with their varied cultures, as containing potential for conflict at many levels. He was particularly concerned with the resolution of cultural conflicts between East and West. He characterized this as a contrast between "esthetics in the East" and "science in the West." His hope was for "a more inclusive truly international cultural ideal which would provide scientifically grounded intellectual and emotional foundations for a partial world sovereignty."

The traditional culture of the Orient, as Professor Northrop commented, is extremely complex, and exceedingly old. Chinese civilization dates from 2852 B.C. Indian culture is based on the *Upanishads* and the *Vedas*, sacred writings that are reputed to be as old as 4000 B.C. Certain portions of this knowledge associated with Eastern cultures requires the actual experiencing of it to be known. Western thinking more often is analytical and logically developed. The West values the kind of knowledge obtained from books and texts, in addition to direct experience. Contemplation is less favored by Western scientists compared to the Eastern traditions, in which intuition is accorded a much higher place in the scheme of things. I find it difficult to read and understand all that Northrop was saying as a scholar and professor of philosophy. If I understand him at least partially, he points out the different ways of seeing the universe and all its contents in the East and the West. Confucianism, Taoism, and Buddhism—three major philosophical and religious traditions in China—have contributed a great deal to its culture. I shall not attempt to outline their precepts nor am I a scholar of Chinese thought or life. Nonetheless it is useful to know that in China, the concept of *Qi* or *Ch'i* (pronounced "chee") is central to much of Chinese medicine, and its later applications in Japanese traditional medicine as well. Qi (*Ki* in Japanese) is the life-energy that flows into and throughout an organism while it is alive. In the West the term, bioenergy, has sometimes been used to refer to the "vital force" that is present in living matter, whether plant, animal, or human. This energy is not readily measured by conventional Western scientific instruments, and is not presently included as a part of acceptable Western science or medicine. This does not keep it from existing, and it has been used as a concept in many practical ways in Eastern medical and healing traditions.

In Traditional Chinese Medicine Qi flows throughout the body in channels that are not blood or lymph vessels but certain pathways called (in translation) "meridians." This is the same term printed on maps, to define latitudes and longitudes. In Chinese medicine there are twelve major meridians, also several hundred lesser ones through which Qi flows. The source of Qi is from the environment, the heavens above and the earth below, and also from food, air and water.

It is a subtle energy that exists in the entire environment. Solar energy is a major source of it as much as more local elements. In India it is called "Prana." The Qi energy is absorbed into the body through openings or portals that are on the skin. These openings are the points referred to as acupuncture points along the meridians. These openings and the meridians have connections deep within the body to all the organ structures.

Another central concept in Chinese philosophy and medicine is the importance of complementary opposites or polarities, called "yin" and "yang" in Chinese. Unlike the Western viewpoint that sees opposites as implying a contest or fight, yin/yang refers to the constant flowing of energy into its opposite. Thus, yin becomes yang, and yang becomes yin. (The only thing constant is change, a Greek philosopher said.) The original meaning of the words was the sunny side and the dark side of a hill. Neither is good or bad, but they have different qualities. Another way of looking at yin and yang is expansion and contraction. This is the basis for the macrobiotic approach to food and nutrition. Foods that create a contraction of energy need to be balanced with foods that expand energy. Eating heavy meats, eggs, and fats produces a contractive tendency in the body and is then balanced by sugars, alcohol, and drugs, for example. In a less severe degree of opposites, leafy vegetables, slightly contractive, balance fruit juices that are defined as expansive. The desired goal of balance in food is reached in macrobiotic nutrition by eating foods more fully balanced in themselves such as grains and vegetables. Thus they require less of other foods to create balance.

Chinese medicine is far more complex than what I have touched on. Health still depends on the correct balancing of energies. Illness is defined as a disharmony or imbalance of energetic forces. Acupuncture is a major treatment method in classical or traditional Chinese medicine for the reestablishment of energy balance in the bodily systems and total organism.

The method of inserting fine needles into specific sites along the meridians to stimulate or dampen the Qi is many centuries old. The needles as used in modern China and throughout the world, including the United States, are very thin that rarely cause any pain, nor do they cause any bleeding if inserted properly in the traditionally defined acupuncture points.

The twelve major meridians are named after major organs, such as the Heart Meridian and the Gallbladder Meridian. This does not mean that the meridian goes only to the specific organ in the body, but that it travels along a set pathway and does involve the functions and activities of the organ for which it is named. The energy of the particular meridian is not limited to the functions of the one organ.

The American Medical Association has called acupuncture and other traditional Chinese medical treatments "experimental" from a Western viewpoint. Being in use five thousand years does not qualify it for acceptance through seniority. There is an American Academy of Medical Acupuncture that trains physicians in acupuncture. It is still not a common method of treatment by M. D.s. There are more non-medical licensed acupuncturists in the United States than physician-acupuncturists. Nineteen states have licensing laws, or a registration of acupuncturists. In some states there are no specific laws regulating it. A few states permit only M. D.s to practice acupuncture. A few insurance companies will reimburse for treatment with acupuncture. It is useful to some extent in the treatment of alcoholism and cocaine addiction, especially when combined with other methods.

Traditional Chinese physicians diagnose in a different way than a Western physician. By a variety of methods they decide if a meridian is underenergized or overenergized. Acupuncture can increase energy in the system or decrease it. It also can "tonify" or balance the energy. One method for determining which meridians are "off" is by pulse diagnosis. This is different from conventional pulse examination. In Chinese medicine and physiology there are twelve different pulses, detected by feeling the pulses at the right and left wrist. Instead of feeling only one pulse, a Chinese traditional doctor feels three pulses lightly at each wrist by placing three fingers at the wrist. Then pressing more firmly and deeply at the same three places on each wrist, three additional pulses are felt on each arm, thus making a total of twelve. The training to detect these twelve pulses is no small feat, and requires several years for proficiency. Each of the separate pulses relates to a different meridian. The quality and sensation of the pulse can be used to diagnose problems in the meridians, and therefore helps establish a diagnosis. Pulse diagnosis by itself is not enough to make a complete diagnosis.

Careful observation of the complexion, face and tongue are also used to a much greater degree than in Western medicine. The oldest Chinese medical textbook is the *Nei Ching,* a book whose title is translated as *The Yellow Emperor's Classic of Internal Medicine* (Veith, 1972). It describes in detail how to examine a patient. It also introduces the idea of psychosomatic illnesses with the statement: "We must know how to determine whether a disorder is caused by perverse energy coming from outside or by emotional stress. Psychological disturbances, like perverse energies, can give rise to muscular disorders and all sorts of illnesses. If psychological disturbances, caused by emotional shocks persist, no treatment can be given, because the mind must be at peace in order for the defensive energy to function properly." The perverse energies are wind, cold, humidity, heat, dryness and fire. The *Nei Ching* —it's full title is *Huang Ti Nei Ching Su Wen*—consists largely of questions and answers between the emperor and his chief minister, Ch'i Po. Some of it reads like the latest guide to health maintenance for the 1990s.

In the beginning of the text the emperor says: "I have heard that in ancient times the people lived through the years to be over a hundred years, and yet they remained active and did not become decrepit in their activities. But nowadays people reach only half of that age and yet become decrepit and failing. Is it because the world changes from generation to generation? Or is it that mankind is becoming negligent of the laws of nature?" (Veith, 1972).

Ch'i Po, the minister, continues to stress the importance of psychological factors. "Before beginning acupuncture treatment, the physician must be well aware of the role of the mental . . . Excessive worry harms the mind. Disorders impair vitality; too much pleasure may dissipate the mind, anxiety may hinder the circulation of energy, anger may lead to death, fear may cause insanity. If the heart has too many worries or wastes away, the complexion deteriorates. A patient afflicted with too many worries will die in winter. The acupuncturist must clearly understand these ideas of the mind and the soul."

This recommendation is as correct today as it was over four thousand years ago. The role of emotions and mental stress is still barely given more than lip service by most conventional physicians in the treatment of physical diseases. Much of this persistent attitude is not primarily an individual trait but more to do with the limited amount of training in present-day medical schools for counseling patients with physical illnesses. The specific pattern of present-day practice in most industrialized countries, especially the United States, also contributes to a lack of close attention to the emotional elements in physical illness. The amount of time spent with each patient keeps shrinking to an assembly-line pattern. With less and less time spent, knowledge of the patient as a person is not easily gained. Even specialists may spend as little as five or ten minutes with patients unless there is a complicated diagnostic problem.

The experience of James Reston, newspaper correspondent for the *New York Times,* created a significant increase of interest in Chinese medicine in the United States. In 1971 Reston accompanied President Nixon on his trip to China. Reston required an emergency appendectomy, which was carried out using acupuncture anesthesia. Both Richard Nixon and James Reston contributed to a meeting of East and West in their own ways. For more than twenty years since then, there has been an expanding attention to Chinese medicine in the United States.

When Chairman Mao became the head of the Chinese government in 1949, a decision was made to allow traditional Chinese medicine to be offered to the citizens of China along with Western-type medical care. At that time there were fifteen thousand modern doctors and five hundred thousand traditional ones.

There are now many schools of traditional Chinese medicine in existence as well as Western, or modern, types. In 1955 the Central Bureau of Hygiene of the Chinese government reformed medical education. They decreed at the same time that traditional Chinese medicine was to be taught on an equal footing with techniques borrowed from the West. A Chinese Academy of Traditional Medicine was created in Beijing, with institutes in the provinces. There are also combinations of both systems, as was true of James Reston's appendectomy.

Traditional Chinese medicine is not a unified or single body of knowledge. The older way of training was for a student to work under a master for many years in an apprenticeship, similar to the training of nineteenth century American physicians. In the early 1960s the Chinese government brought together a group of acceptable Chinese physicians who were asked to formulate what constituted "Traditional Chinese Medicine." The result was a semi-standardized set of methods that were then to be taught to the Chinese people and to foreigners. This produced a more rigid version that left out many variations.

In the United States today there are colleges of Oriental or Chinese traditional medicine. Some Americans have studied in China and Macao (near Hongkong), and have completed the four to five years required to obtain the degree of O. M. D., or Doctor of Oriental Medicine. Until recently the director of the Pain and Stress Relief Clinic at the Lemuel Shattuck Hospital in Boston, Massachusetts was Ted J. Kaptchuk, O. M. D. For anyone interested in a clear understanding of Chinese medicine Dr. Kaptchuk's *The Web That Has No Weaver* (Kaptchuk, 1983) gives an excellent presentation of the theory and practice of Chinese medicine. As a comment on the cover states: "An American fully trained in the practice of Chinese medicine explains this 'nonscientific' but often astoundingly effective system of healing."

In the early 1970s, a few years after acupuncture was having some impact in the United States due to James Reston's experience, new programs for training both medical and non-M. D. acupuncturists came into existence. At that time I heard a lecture at a medical society meeting by a professor of psychiatry, an expert on hypnosis. He challenged the concepts of Chinese medicine and acupuncture by pointing out what he considered proof that it was "nothing more than hypnosis." At the time I was not aware, nor did anyone in the audience raise the issue, that acupuncture has been used extensively in veterinary medicine on horses, cows, and dogs. These animals are not usually known to be suggestible nor readily hypnotizable.

It may be of interest that the first person credited with performing hypnosis in Western countries was Franz Mesmer of Austria in the late 1700s. He called his methods "magnetic healing," since he thought that magnets were a necessary part of the procedure. Later, in the nineteenth century, the explanation for hypnosis included several theories relating to energy flow throughout the body. Mesmer's work was discredited, but some of his techniques later developed into hypnosis. In the 1840s in India a British surgeon, James Esdaile, M. D., was able to perform over one hundred surgical operations using hypnosis. Since anesthesia had been discovered at the same time, with the use of chloroform, Esdaile's work was easily ignored. I raise the question: might hypnosis be a special Western form of energy healing that in some way taps into the same Qi energy that the Chinese have dealt with for centuries? This is highly speculative but at least it could be a rebuttal by some Chinese physicians who might see some of the Western world's concepts as too narrow and limiting.

There has been research with radioactive isotopes that would appear to prove the existence of the meridian pathways. A researcher injected small amounts of radioactive isotopes into acupuncture points and could measure that the material was absorbed, while injections just outside the acupuncture points showed no absorption. There also are instruments that can be used to find acupuncture points. The instrument looks somewhat like a pocket flashlight but has a galvanometer that measures skin resistance. When it is passed slowly over an acupuncture point the instrument shows a drop in electrical potential. The points thus located match the traditional Chinese locations that have been established over the centuries.

Treatment methods in traditional Chinese medicine also include moxibustion, which makes use of the acupuncture points without any needling. Instead a small cone made from certain herbs is placed on the skin and ignited so that the heat penetrates the skin at the acupuncture point without burning the skin. The most common herb used for moxibustion is Artemesia or Mugwort. Mugwort is only one of thousands of herbs that are a common part of Chinese medicine. A visit to a Chinese pharmacy in China or in some Chinatowns of American cities would reveal hundreds of bottles of herbal preparations. Some of these combine six or eight different herbs.

Dietary guidance is an essential part of Chinese medical treatment, with the goal of restoring harmony and balance to the total person: mind, body and spirit. Exercises of various kinds are used both for prevention and treatment. One type that has become well-known in other countries of the world, including the United States, is T'ai Chi. A Chinese T'ai Chi master, Cheng Man-Ching came to the United States several decades ago and taught American students his form of T'ai Chi. As a young man Cheng had contracted tuberculosis and was not expected to live. Through the use of T'ai Chi, he fully recovered and lived to his seventies. Several of his students in turn became teachers and taught in New Haven, Connecticut. I had the opportunity to participate in one of his students' classes for a year when I lived in Connecticut.

T'ai Chi looks like slow-motion ballet with vigorous body control coupled with breathing. To learn it requires the careful copying and practicing of highly specific movements of the arms, legs, torso and chest. I did not become proficient at it due to lack of discipline in practicing it regularly.

Travelogues of China frequently show pictures of large groups of Chinese citizens of all ages doing T'ai Chi outdoors as a morning exercise. A complete set of thirty-eight connected positions can take about twenty minutes. There is a careful emphasis on connecting the breathing with the movements, and maintaining proper balance at the same time. Paradoxically it is slow and calm in movement and yet can produce strength and energy. It is not usually a martial arts defense and attack system, but it has been used occasionally for that purpose as well.

Massage is also known and practiced within traditional Chinese medicine. One type is a massage of the acupuncture points. If the massage is done with the pressure of the fingernail in a clockwise direction, it is considered "tonifying" or increasing the energy. If done in a counterclockwise direction, it is sedating. Another more generalized type of massage is called *amma*. This has been defined by Michio Kushi (Kushi, 1991) as "a physically-oriented application for stiff joints and muscles, and problems caused by stagnation in the circulation of blood and energy." It has much in common with Western forms of massage.

A more recently popularized development in China that has also been imported to the United States is *Qi Gong*. It dates from 2500 B.C. It is a deep breathing exercise that teaches the use of Qi, or energy. A Qi Gong master teaches the students to use "internal Qi" on themselves. There is also "external Qi," which can produce an effect on others. Advanced Qi Gong masters are reported to be capable to move inanimate objects without touching them directly. It has also been stated that they can shrink cancer cells in test tubes, and heal animals with Qi Gong. In some public gatherings in China some of the effects are thought to be partly a matter of suggestion.

A detailed description of feats by Qi Gong masters was reported by David Eisenberg, M. D. in *Encounters with Qi* (Eisenberg,1987). Dr. Eisenberg described his year in China in 1979 as the first American medical exchange student to the People's Republic of China. He reports that millions of cancer patients in China practice Qi Gong. There are many forms of Qi Gong numbering about four hundred. The claims are that they raise resistance to disease, and aid in healing.

Chinese medicine can qualify as a truly holistic system, since it does not separate the person and his body from mind and spirit. It is as much a psychotherapy as a physical therapy, in concept and in practice. It resembles homeopathy in its looking very closely at the individual who has the illness more than the disease as a separate entity. Hippocrates similarly said, "It is more important to know the person who has the disease than the disease the person has."

Leon Hammer, M. D. is an unusual American physician who trained and has practiced as a psychiatrist, psychoanalyst, and child psychiatrist for more than twenty-five years. He also studied Chinese medicine for at least twelve years and has practiced it more than seventeen years. He has written a detailed exposition of Chinese medicine, *Dragon Rises, Red Bird Flies* (Hammer, 1990), which elaborates the holistic aspects of Chinese medicine clearly. Although much of the text is technical and specialized, several chapters give a highly readable presentation of what he has learned and observed from patients and from his education. In his chapter on "A Medical Model" he comments:

Humanistic psychology seeks a congenial medical model within which it can function without conflict. I believe Chinese medicine is a medical system with which Western psychology is highly congruent. Chinese medicine is a medicine-philosophy. In ideology and methodology it considers man in dynamic interplay with his total environment.

As a form of medicine it contributes to a unified concept of human life, within each person and with the entire universe. Chinese medicine embodies a remarkable union of technical competence and spiritual force. Because it is also a successful method of alleviating suffering, Chinese medicine may succeed in bringing popular attention to the unifying concepts of the East more quickly and completely than any other manifestation of Oriental thought.

The term, Oriental medicine, at times may appear to be identical to Chinese medicine. This is not entirely accurate since there are medical traditions and practices in other countries that are also many centuries old, in Korea, Japan, and India. Some of China's culture derives from India, as was also true that some of Japan's culture derived from China. In the period of the sixth and seventh century A. D. many of China's religious teachings, medical practices and writings were brought back to Japan by Japanese emissaries to China and Korea. The distinct Japanese culture modified and adapted these over the following centuries. The Japanese term for a traditional form of medical practice is *Kampo*. There is a revival of interest and practice of traditional medicine in Japan today in Kampo, which means "Chinese method."

10

Japanese Medicine: Kampo and Other Approaches

Japan has maintained its own distinct values and traditions dating back to the beginning centuries of its civilization. These have been preserved to the present day, despite the extensive industrialization of Japan in the past thirty-five years. Japan had also absorbed certain elements of Western culture during the sixteenth, nineteenth and twentieth centuries. A few elements of Japan's culture and traditions are derived from Chinese influences in the sixth and seventh centuries. The history of present-day Japanese medicine begins in the sixth and seventh centuries A. D. when Buddhism was brought from China along with Chinese medical concepts and practices.

Before this time there were a few other contacts from outside Japan. A Korean physician arrived in 414 A. D. In 561 A. D. Chi Chung, a physician from southern China, brought more than a hundred books on theoretical medicine to Japan. In 593 A. D. the Japanese empress, Suiko, sent armies to Korea where Chinese medicine was already established. As a result of this contact representatives from Japan went to China. In the next two centuries Chinese Buddhists arrived in Japan (Lock, 1980).

As early as 702 A. D. the ruling government in Japan authorized a ministry of health, under the Taiho code of governmental procedures. By 900 A. D. a variety of medical systems had been established. Buddhist monks conducted much of medical practice and they established the first hospitals. Acupuncture, moxibustion (kyu), massage (amma), and herbal medicine were major forms of treatment, derived from Chinese Traditional Medicine. Until 1000 A. D. all written material in Japan was in Chinese. Japanese printing and writing today is derived from Chinese script or ideograms.

Kampo: Many Chinese herbs and plant materials could not be cultivated in Japan due to climatic differences. Some limitation on the spread of Chinese herbal medicine also existed due to lack of raw materials. Trade, therefore, had to be established between China and Japan to import herbs for Japan. There were other reasons as well for establishing trade. The Japanese term, Kampo referred to Chinese medicine, since the word literally means "the Chinese method." Today in modern Japan Kampo medicine refers only to the use of herbs and not the other features of Chinese medicine, such as acupuncture, moxibustion and massage.

Qi, or Ki in Japanese, is central to Japanese traditional medicine, as in Chinese medicine. Also Taoist philosophy and some derivatives of Confucianism have been absorbed into some of the earlier practices of Japanese traditional medicine. In an excellent study of traditional Kampo medicine in present-day Japan, *East Asian Medicine in Urban Japan* (Lock, 1980) the author refers to the medical beliefs and practices of China, Korea and Japan until the nineteenth century as "East Asian medicine" in contrast to Western or modern medicine, which she calls "cosmopolitan" medicine. These two systems exist today in Japan and China, both separately and combined in Japan.

A second cultural "invasion" occurred in Japan in the sixteenth century with the arrival of Portuguese and Dutch traders. This led to the introduction of "modern" medicine. During the Azuchi-Momoyama period of 1569–1600, Buddhism was oppressed. Traditional medicine continued on a more nonreligious basis. One leader, Dosan Manase, established the "Goseiha" school of traditional medicine, highly abstract and theoretical in its writings, but practical in action, according to Margaret Lock (Lock, 1980). The art of mixing several herbs and substances, as many as twenty, was perfected, although the portions of mixtures used were small.

About one hundred years later "Kohoha," another school of traditional medicine was established, which emphasized a return to the classic Chinese texts of medicine. A Chinese book from 200 A. D. was the basis for this school. The text in Chinese was *Shang Han Lun*, or *Shokanron* in Japanese. It emphasized the principle that the course of disease, especially fevers, characteristically had six stages. The correct treatment depended on determination of which stage the illness had reached. Emphasis was more on treatment than theory, and the number of medications was more limited than the Goseiha school. These schools contributed to the later modern forms of traditional East Asian medicine in Japan (Lock, 1980).

As part of the Kohoha tradition Todo Yoshimasu (1720–1773) developed a highly complex technique of abdominal palpation, which is still used by some present-day Kampo physicians. With the arrival of the Dutch a school of medicine known as "Rangaku" evolved. This stressed practicality and less theoretical speculation. Surgical techniques were included, but the older Chinese traditions were maintained for non-surgical problems. Only the wealthier citizens, aristocrats, and samurai had access to the licensed doctors. For the remainder of the population unlicensed doctors practiced a blend of Kampo and folk medicine (Lock, 1980).

Before 1600 most physicians learned massage, or amma, but in later generations this became more for relaxation and enjoyment, and not for treatment. The custom grew for blind persons to administer massage. Official examinations were established with graded levels of ability. Fees were based on the level of ability. Some blind massagers also learned acupuncture. Eventually this led to both massage and acupuncture losing some of its prestige, since the blind had a lower social status. Gradually the higher class urban physicians limited their practice to herbal medicine, without any massage, and a lesser amount of acupuncture and moxibustion.

In 1824 the Rangaku (Dutch-influenced) school introduced smallpox vaccination. This further weakened the more traditional Kampo physicians (Lock, 1980). Still greater challenges by Western medicine arrived within forty years, when Admiral Perry of the United States Navy sailed to Japan in 1858 and Japan was forced to open its borders to the influence of the West. German physicians arrived shortly afterward. By 1869 the Japanese government officially adopted the German system of medicine and medical education. In 1873 there still were twenty-three thousand Kampo doctors and only five hundred and twenty registered M.D.s. This changed rapidly. In 1876 a law was passed in Japan that all physicians had to study Western medicine. Kampo was not outlawed but discouraged. By 1883 regulations restricted the practice of Kampo more severely. Many Kampo physicians became pharmacists and continued to administer herbal preparations (Lock, 1980).

The period of 1868 to 1912 was known as the Meiji era. During this time Western medicine, and many elements of Western culture, art and nutrition were introduced. Separate from the now Westernized medical training and practice, the government created schools for acupuncture, moxibustion and massage, without the use of medications, herbal or modern. In 1973 there were forty thousand registered practitioners of acupuncture, moxibustion and massage. The training requires three years followed by a state examination for licensure. The number of M.D.s today in Japan is about one hundred and seventy thousand in a country of one hundred twenty million.

Because of the Russo-Japanese War of 1904–1905, the treatment of war injuries and the use of surgery fully established the place of modern medicine in Japan. Kampo medicine did not disappear but faded into the background. From 1934 to 1945 a Kampo Medicine Association was created but then dissolved. In 1938 an East Asian Medical Organization was created, and published a monthly *Clinical Kampo Journal*.

Still later an active revival of Kampo medicine began, referred to by the Japanese press as "Kampo Boomu," or the Kampo Boom. In 1976 the Japanese government passed a law allowing certain herbal prescriptions—more than one hundred—to be acceptable under the National Health Insurance system. A leading newspaper called the event, "Kampo Gannen," the first year of the reign of Kampo.

Mr. Akira Tsumura reports in his recently published book on Kampo medicine, *Kampo: How the Japanese Updated Traditional Herbal Medicine* (Tsumura, 1991) that 42.7 percent of the M. D.s of Japan prescribe some Kampo medicines. There are some physicians who specialize in Kampo and are directors of small Kampo clinics, which include both inpatient and outpatient treatments. Mr. Tsumura points out that the art of Kampo healing is based on the principle that the human organism poseses the inherent ability to protect, regulate and heal itself. Mr. Tsumura himself is the director of a large manufacturing company that produces herbal or Kampo medications using modern methods for extraction and quality control. Research is also carried out to find the best combinations, and also find new substances that have therapeutic value.

Tsumura lists in detail more than forty unrefined herbs that have medicinal value, with their chemical constituents, their pharmacological properties, and their usage according to Japanese classic writings. He also names and describes Kampo preparations that use the unrefined substances. He lists in detail the composition of about eighty Kampo preparations, which can be obtained in capsule form. The traditional herbal mixtures required the patient to brew a tea from the several herbs that were in a preparation. An example of a commonly used Kampo preparation as described by Mr. Tsumura is *Sho-saiko-to*. He gives the following data about it:

Efficacy:

Used for those with an average constitution who have discomfort and distention of the upper abdomen, tongue fur, unpleasant feeling in the mouth, loss of appetite, nausea, and may occasionally have low grade fever with the following illnesses: Various febrile diseases, pneumonia, bronchitis, colds, pleurisy, tuberculosis, lymphangitis, chronic complaints of the digestive system, liver complaints, incomplete recovery from child birth.

Ingredients:

Bupleuri Radix (ChineseThoroughwax)	7.0 grams
Pinelliae Tuber	5.0
Scutellariae Radix (Baical Skullcap)	3.0
Zizyphi Fructus (Giant Jujube tree fruit)	3.0
Ginseng Radix	3.0
Glycyrrhizae Radix (Chinese licorice)	2.0
Zingisberis Rhizoma (ginger)	1.0

Usage-SHO:

Used for those with an average constitution with tenderness and distension of the hypochondrium.

1) Febrile diseases accompanied with a loss of appetite, unpleasant feeling in the mouth, etc.
2) Various chronic diseases that are accompanied with tenderness and distention of the hypochondrium.
3) Various chronic diseases that are accompanied with a loss of appetite, fatigue, etc.
4) Strengthens children with weak constitutions.

In this Kampo preparation seven different herbs have been combined in the proportions listed. A sample description of one of the ingredients, Zizyphi fructus, or fruit of the Jujube tree, in the text is as follows:

Jujube (Fruit)

Rhamnaceae, *Zizyphus jujuba MILL. var. inermis REHD. Common name: Jujube, Red Dat, Ziziphus*
Japanese pronunciation: Taiso
Background: Herbal healers throughout the Far East from China to Malaysia are familiar with this herb. Traditionally, it is considered to have an affinity for the heart, spleen, liver and gall-bladder. It is used as a sedative to the liver, a cardiotonic, and to treat insomnia and cold sweats.

KAMPO: The fruit is used (Zizyphi Fructus)

Main Constituents: Triterpine: oleanolic acid, butulinic acid, alphitolic acid and p-croumaric esters, ursolic acid. Saponins: zizyphus saponin. Others: sugars, malic acid, tartaric acid, clyclic AMP, cyclic GMP.

Pharmacological properties: Anti-allergic, anti-peptic ulcer, anti-stress.

Usage according to Japanese classics: Used mainly to treat severe cramps. Also relieves coughing, severe palpitations that seem to rise upward in the body, discomfort, pain and abdominal pain

Used in Kampo prescriptions:
Irei-To, Eppi-Ka-Jutsu-To, Ogi-Kenchu-To, Oren-To,
Kakkon-To, Sho-Saiko-To (and 31 other Kampo mixtures)

There are now three research centers in Japan devoted entirely to research on medicinal herbs, and for the purpose of examining tropical plants for their medicinal value. According to Akira Tsumura, Kampo preparations may help to cure many chronic diseases still considered incurable in conventional medical thinking, such as those associated with aging. They also can counteract the side-effects of many new drugs. Tsumura refers to the World Health Organization's call for a "New Medicine" that can combine the best of the scientific world with as much of traditional systems of medicine as can be properly regulated and combined with specific national health systems.

Since 1980 there has been a *Chinese Journal of Integrated Traditional and Western Medicine.* Japan has been able over the centuries to absorb other traditions and cultures' ideas and practices without abandoning their own viewpoint. The revival of Kampo medicine is an example of this type of blending. There are plans for some Kampo preparations to be introduced into the United States within the next few years. It will be interesting to see if American medicine also can consider the use of herbal preparations that have been carefully prepared with the use of high-tech processes.

It may be necessary that these preparations would be sold over-the-counter. This is now the practice with European herbs and other plant materials that are not rated as acceptable as medication by the Food and Drug Administration or the medical profession. Perhaps in exchange for what the West has given or taught to the Japanese, they can reciprocate in both a technological and a traditional way, by encouraging some of the ancient practices of Kampo medicine.

MASSAGE: Some elements of Japanese massage have been derived from Chinese "amma" methods, which eventually were applied more for relaxation and pleasure and less as a treatment method. There are reportedly over two hundred and fifty different schools of massage in Japan, most of them established by the 1850s, by the end of the Edo period. After the Meiji period began in 1868, a therapeutic type of massage developed called *shiatsu* or finger-pressure massage. This was a form of massage applied at the acupuncture points, with techniques of a thrusting and pressing style. The amma methods typically used rubbing techniques. Influences from the West later included chiropractic elements, especially in Kyoto and Osaka, with increased emphasis on the spine, and some decrease in attention to traditional methods. Still later and into the present era, Western styles of massage were introduced, with emphasis on muscle tissue and less on pressure points. Advertisements for "massaji" emphasized relaxation instead of therapy. Shiatsu, however, is still considered a therapeutic technique. This does not prevent so-called relaxation types of massage, whether in Japan or in the United States, from being health-enhancing and therapeutic as well.

MACROBIOTICS: The meeting of East and West continues to be a cyclic process back and forth over the centuries and the decades. Although the development and elaboration of macrobiotics was first developed in Japan by Yukikazu Sakurazawa, also known as George Ohsawa, it has not been a significant part of mainstream Japanese culture. Ohsawa did derive some ideas from Sagen Ishizuka, a Western-trained physician during the first decades of the modernization of Japan.

Dr. Ishizuka became interested in the role of nutrition in disease, and wrote a book in 1897 outlining his theories of nutrition. His ideas were not accepted by most Japanese physicians, then trained mostly in the Western tradition of Germany. This is similar to the situation today in the United States for many physicians who speak out for a larger role for nutrition as a cause and as a treatment of many diseases.

Ohsawa lived in France and the United States for a portion of his life, besides Japan. After traveling and living in several countries of the world, George Ohsawa returned to Japan and began teaching about macrobiotics, the word he chose to give to his ideas. The word itself had been coined much earlier by a German physician, Wilhelm von Hufeland, in 1796. He wrote a book, *Makrobiotik oder die Kunst das menschliche Leben zu Verlangern,* or "Macrobiotics, or the Art of Prolonging Life." Von Hufeland had been the personal physician of the famous German writer, Goethe.

Ohsawa emphasized a return to the more traditional diet of Japan at a time when Japan was moving in the opposite direction, eating more Western-style foods, including more meat, dairy, and sugar. Since the end of World War II Japan has become even more Americanized in its eating habits. Visitors to Japan who have revisited in recent years after a period of twenty to thirty years have told me that Japanese schoolchildren physically appear heavier and more obese than they looked thirty years ago. Some aspects of American and Western culture may be a mixed blessing for the Japanese as well as for Americans themselves.

At Ohsawa's suggestion and encouragement, one of his disciples, Michio Kushi, came to the United States in 1949. He has become a major force in not only the development of the "Macrobiotic Movement" but has had an influence on the entire natural foods and whole foods industry. Michio Kushi started Erewhon, one of the first natural foods companies, and founded the East West Foundation and its Journal. Both Erewhon and the *East West Journal* are now independent of Michio Kushi, but were strongly shaped by him.

Another leader in the macrobiotic movement is Herman Aihara, now in Oroville, California, where he is the director of the Vega Center. He has been a writer and teacher about macrobiotics for several decades. Other Japanese disciples of Ohsawa came to the United States over a period of years. Michio Kushi has developed macrobiotics to the point that it is now a worldwide movement. After Ohsawa's death in 1965, some of his followers continued in Japan on a small scale to teach and practice his ideas about health and nutrition. In 1980 a macrobiotic center was opened in Tokyo by an American, Phillip Jannetta, and his Japanese wife. Jannetta had trained under Michio Kushi for several years. What had originated in Japan has been brought back to Japan partly by Americans. It still remains a small movement, but may have greater impact in coming years, as the Japanese join Americans to look at the evidence that supports the role of nutrition in maintaining health and for the treatment of illness.

Japan derived some of its traditional and present-day medical practices from both China earlier and from the West beginning in the nineteenth century. China in turn derived some of its earliest medical concepts and practices from India, the land of an ancient civilization, now five thousand years old, and still very much alive and growing.

11
Ayurvedic Medicine: Old and New

Few Americans or Europeans would be likely to recognize the word, *Ayurveda,* unless they happened to be scholars or had spent several months in India. This had been true until a little over a decade ago, when Ayurvedic knowledge moved from East to West, with the arrival of Dr. Vasant Lad, an Ayurvedic physician. Ayurveda means "the science of life and longevity" in Sanskrit, the ancient language of India. The name of the most ancient scriptures of the Hindu tradition are the Vedas, estimated to be five thousand years old.

Ayurveda refers to those scriptures that deal with health and healing. Originally, they were passed from generation to generation from memory, until they were finally written down more than two thousand years ago. They formed the basis for the medical and healing practices throughout India not only in ancient times but continuously into the present.

India is a large country, sometimes called a subcontinent, with people speaking many languages, practicing many religions, living in a range of climates and cultures. The earliest evidence of human village life in the world was discovered through excavations in the Indus River valley. The cities of Harappa and Mohenjo-daro are five thousand years old. The original inhabitants were dark-skinned Dravidians, who later were invaded by lighter-skinned people from the northwest and west, from what is now Afghanistan and possibly Persia. In later centuries Darius, King of Persia, brought his influence into India in 800 B. C. Later Alexander the Great of Macedonia extended his empire in 300 B. C. with marches into western India. Many centuries later in the eighth and ninth centuries A. D., the Islamic Moguls came to rule in India. In l498 Vasco da Gama of Portugal arrived on the Malabar coast and established contact between Europe and India. By 1600 the British arrived with the East India Company taking control of much of India until the final independence of India in 1947.

Throughout these centuries Ayurveda evolved as a system of health maintenance and medical/surgical treatment. The two earliest texts of medicine were written in the first and second centuries A. D. The first was a medical text, *Charaka Samhita*, named after a famous Ayurvedic physician, Charaka, considered the father of medicine in India, comparable to Hippocrates for the West. The second text, *Sushruta Samhita,* dealt mainly with surgery. Additional classics were written several centuries later. As Hindu culture itself was carried to other countries, Ayurveda also was brought to Indonesia in the East, to Tibet, and to the West where it had some influence on ancient Greek medicine. Later, as Buddhism grew out of Hinduism in India and then was brought to Sri Lanka, Burma and other Buddhist lands, including China, Ayurveda was also brought to these lands. An outstanding Buddhist sage, Nagarjuna of the Mahayana Buddhist tradition, was an Ayurvedic doctor.

In 1833 the British East India Company had sufficient authority and control to close and ban all Ayurvedic schools. The first university for Western medicine was then opened in Calcutta. This relegated Ayurvedic medicine to rural areas, and for those who could not afford Western medicine. Ayurveda obviously lost much of its earlier prestige and became mixed with folk medicine. With the establishment of India's independence in 1947, Ayurvedic medical schools regained official acceptance. Now there are one hundred Ayurvedic medical schools, requiring five to six years of training, and one hundred Western medical schools.

My personal interest in India and its culture began as an adolescent when I enjoyed going to an Indian restaurant in New York City. I also had the experience of hearing and seeing a dance and music concert by Uday Shankar, older brother of Ravi Shankar, a famous present-day Indian musician. Yet, I had not known anything about Ayurveda until three years ago. I then discovered that Ayurveda was not only an interesting expression of the culture of India in past centuries and practiced as folk medicine. It also has relevance for present-day life in the United States and throughout the world.

In 1983 the World Health Organization held a conference in Alma Ata, U.S.S.R. about medical care in developing countries. Ayurveda was seen as a most helpful and practical system to consider, applicable to any climate, and capable of being used self-supportively, because of its great emphasis on prevention. Increasingly it is now being studied and practiced in the United States, India, and other countries as a part of modern medical care.

All this has been happening at an accelerating rate. I have not investigated the entire scope of its practice in the United States, but I have became familiar with several people and centers that have been presenting the principles and practices of Ayurvedic medicine over the past decade.

Dr. Vasant Lad, a native of India, came to the United States in 1979 after he had been a Professor of Clinical Medicine at Poona University College of Ayurvedic Medicine for fifteen years. He had also served for three years as Medical Director of the Ayurvedic Hospital in Poona. In 1981 he established a fulltime program of study on Ayurveda at The Ayurvedic Institute in Albuquerque and Santa Fé, New Mexico. He has lectured and trained students in several other parts of the United states, including Boston, Massachusetts. He has summarized his views on Ayurveda in *Ayurveda: The Science of*

Self-Healing (Lad, 1984). He wrote a second book, *The Yoga of Herb*s written in 1986 with Dr. David Frawley of Santa Fé, New Mexico (Frawley & Lad, 1986).

Dr. Frawley is an American who has an O. M. D. degree (Doctor of Oriental Medicine) from the International Institute of Chinese Medicine and has practiced herbal medicine extensively. He is one of the few Westerners to be recognized in India as an authentic teacher of the ancient Vedic wisdom. He has written a comprehensive guide to Ayurvedic medicine, *Ayurvedic Healing* (Frawley, 1989). It is an attempt to convey in modern terms the traditions of Ayurveda.

I had the opportunity to hear Dr. Vasant Lad speak and teach in Boston in 1991 at The Ayurvedic Rehabilitation Center. He is an excellent teacher who demonstrates thorough knowledge of his subject. At the same time he also conveys an essential element of Ayurveda, its spiritual element, that is interwoven with the physical and mental/emotional aspects of the teaching. Ayurveda is a holistic system of medicine, since it actively concerns itself with mind, body and spirit. It does not make a clear separation between mind and body, and considers the spiritual element as undergirding the other two.

The first American to graduate with a degree from an Indian school of Ayurvedic medicine is Dr. Robert Svoboda. He was a student of Dr. Vasant Lad in Poona, India at the Tilak Ayurveda Mahavidhyalaya Medical School. Dr. Svoboda graduated in 1980. Since then he has traveled extensively in the U.S. and Canada, lecturing and conducting workshops. He has written several books on Ayurvedic medicine. His most recent, *Prakuti: Your Ayurvedic Constitution* (Svoboda, 1989) is an excellent introduction to the subject.

Another example of modern-day interest and application of Ayurveda is presented by a Viennese pharmacist, Birgit Heyn, in her book, *Ayurveda: The Indian Art of Natural Medicine and Life Extension* (Heyn, 1983). She became disenchanted with conventional medicine and the overdependency of patients on synthetic drugs. She studied Ayurveda at the Hindu University of Benares, and also with other Indian teachers.

The Ayurvedic approach to the treatment of a person is highly individualized. It is the person who is treated more than the disease. This is in contrast to conventional medicine, which diagnoses the disease and treats accordingly but with only slight adjustment to the specific person being treated. An essential element of Ayurveda is the determination of the constitutional body/mind type. This classification of types is called *Doshas,* which are established genetically at the time of conception, according to Ayurveda. There are three primary types, called *Vata, Pitta* and *Kapha.* These terms have characteristics that describe the body, the personality, and many other qualities of bodily functioning. The dosha determines which kinds of diet, exercise, and medical therapies are appropriate or contraindicated. Knowing one's own body type is also of importance to a person for better understanding of self. There is no clear separation of body and mind, so the term, bodymind, also could be used. Every mental action has a corresponding event in the body. This ancient belief is now being documented in the scientific laboratories throughout the world, including the National Institute of Mental Health and National Institutes of Health in Washington. The field of psychoneuroimmunology has been repeatedly proving this truth.

The doshas can be combined into subtypes. There are ten different combinations. The three primary doshas are associated with basic psycho-physiological processes of the organism. Vata controls movement. Pitta controls metabolism, and Kapha controls structure. As in Chinese and Japanese traditional medicine, the central principle for health is the proper balancing of energy. The Chinese and Japanese have called this energy Qi or Ki. In the Hindu tradition and in Ayurveda the term for this universal and personal energy is "prana." In Sanskrit, "pra" means "first unit" and "na" means "energy." This is similar to the "Vital Force" that Samuel Hahnemann described in his development of homeopathy. None of these ideas of a generalized bio-energy has ever met with wide acceptance by Western science.

Prana is not just a physical energy but is also a mental energy. Western science has tended to break phenomena into pieces in order to analyze. Eastern views are more holistic and intuitive. From a pranic view the physical level is expressed in matter and the mental level by thoughts. There is also a separate energy level, possibly between the two. This viewpoint proposes that one can alter the energy pattern from either the physical level or the mental level. Physical activity such as breathing techniques or physical postures, as in Hatha Yoga, can increase or change the focus of energy that would then change the total energy picture. On the other hand, through the use of mental activities, such as meditation or other mind activities, the total balance of energy also can be changed. In the Indian tradition there are fine pathways of energy that have been mapped out called "nadis" that resemble the Chinese meridians but are more subtle and possibly thinner. It is claimed that there are seventy-two thousand such nadis.

These various pathways converge and have crossroads throughout the body. These centers are called "chakras" and are located along the length of the body. There are usually seven major ones, beginning at the base of the spine and extending upwards to a point outside the body about six or seven inches above the head. This highest one is called the Crown chakra. The lowest chakra is the Root chakra. The second chakra is at the level of the genitals, but is not in the organs or glands, but is associated with them. The third chakra is at the level of the solar plexus in the middle of the abdomen. The fourth chakra is the Heart chakra. The fifth is the Throat chakra, and the sixth is at a point between both eyes but just above them on the brow. This is often called the "third eye" or Brow chakra. The seventh is the Crown chakra.

The psychology and physiology of the chakra system is an intricate one that is worthy of extensive study and has been used for spiritual practices, also having application to a different way of understanding human psychology and behavior. Many Western psychologists have found it useful for a broader understanding of people. Other cultures of the world have independently developed similar systems of thinking. The American Indian totem pole represents the seven chakras in their use of animal carvings for seven energy levels.

When the doshas are all in balance ideally, perfect health is reached and maintained. Many forces, both internal and external, are constantly throwing the energies out of balance. The challenge is to apply various methods to strengthen the weakened doshas or decrease those that are overcharged. It is essential in Ayurveda first to figure out correctly the dosha type, since this is a guide to corrective action.

The Ayurvedically trained physician asks questions to diagnose the dosha pattern of the patient. Another means of diagnosis is observation of the physical and mental characteristics of the patient. As important as knowing the type or subtype that a person is, it is also essential to evaluate the types of imbalances themselves at a particular time. A person may be evaluated as, for example, a Vata-Pitta type in their basic constitution, but they may be out of balance at a particular time in their Kapha dosha, or they may be out of balance in the Pitta dosha, since everyone has within them all three doshas present, despite their constitutional type.

I underwent an Ayurvedic examination a year ago from an American physician who had received training in a short but concentrated program, sufficient to allow the inclusion of some Ayurvedic methods into a conventional general family practice. There are presently two such physicians in Maine, where I live, and another two hundred physicians throughout the United States.

After I answered a questionnaire, which could be used to estimate the proportion of doshas, the physician asked several additional questions, and felt my pulse based on Ayurvedic methods. I was then informed that my dosha constitution was diagnosed as Vata/Pitta. This meant that I had some characteristics associated with Vata and some with Pitta.

Some typical characteristics or qualities associated with the Vata dosha are as follows:

1. Physically often very active
2. Emotional pattern is fearful, insecure, unpredictable
3. Speech fast
4. Mind restless, active
5. Elimination: tends toward constipation
6. Pulse thready, feeble, moves like a snake

(from *Vasant Lad*)

There are many other qualities relating to bodily characteristics, taste preferences, sleep and dream patterns. These all can be used to decide the prevailing doshas. The other primary doshas of Pitta and Kapha have their individual characteristics. When a dual or blended type is diagnosed, as in Vata/Pitta, then the prevailing qualities of both are found, with one somewhat stronger than the other. In listing some qualities found in Pitta, Dr. Robert Svoboda mentions the following:

1. Skin: delicate, irritable, prone to rashes and pimples, and inflammations, in contrast to Vata, which has dry skin.
2. Hair: red hair or light-colored, or grey or white an early age.
3. Appetite: excellent, really enjoy eating; irritable if they fail to eat when hungry.
4. Elimination: rarely constipated
5. Physically active so long as they don't overheat; average muscle tone, better than Vata
6. Pulse: full, regular, strong, jumping like a frog

(from *Robert Svoboda*)

Pitta dosha has other qualities, many relating to heat and warmth of body and personality. Few if any persons fit these descriptions exactly, and some qualities in a particular person may be different from the usual listing. Nonetheless there is a matching that takes place that can be a useful guide for health maintenance to avoid the development of illness, and also as guidelines for the treatment of diseases. The books on Ayurveda give detailed descriptions of the doshas. They also describe methods for treating imbalances once they are properly diagnosed.

Deepak Chopra in *Perfect Health* (Chopra, 1990) points out that Vata imbalance is a common disorder in America. It is not Vata itself that causes problems, but rather Vata imbalance. I am reminded of a book by John W. Farquhar, M. D., titled *The American Way of Life Need Not Be Hazardous to Your Health* (Farquhar, 1978). It need not be, but often *is*, hazardous.

When I underwent the Ayurvedic examination, the doctor took my pulse in a different way than is usual in Western medicine. Instead of the usual single pulse felt at the wrist, three pulses were examined. This is similar to Chinese pulse diagnosis in some respects, except the Ayurvedic system does not directly correlate each pulse to an energy meridian, but relates the quality of the pulses to the doshas. Usually only one wrist is examined in Ayurveda. For men the right wrist pulses are examined and for women the left. Three fingers are placed on the wrist. The first pulse closest to the hand is the Vata pulse. The second next to it is Pitta, and the third is Kapha. Firmer pressure can detect three additional pulses that reflect the constitutional doshas. The qualities of each pulse are compared to what is usually expected. This obviously requires a reasonable amount of practice, but can be learned. The physician who examined me informed me that I was "out of balance" with excess of my Vata and Pitta doshas. (The most experienced Indian Ayurvedic physicians are so skillful that it has been reported or claimed they can detect some of the past history of the patient as well as their present condition.) My Vata-Pitta imbalance meant that I needed to follow recommendations that would help decrease and balance these doshas.

At the conclusion of the examination I was given a detailed computer print-out, which was produced after all the data that had been collected about me had been entered into a specific software program. This was a true blend of the East meeting the West. Some recommendations were simple. When prescribed by a physician, they are likely to have greater impact than merely reading them or hearing them from parents or teachers as a child or later in life. For example, going to bed by ten o'clock to get sufficient rest is not a new scientific discovery. Yet there is no argument against it, other than the pressures that we create for ourselves or are created by our job and culture. Everyone faces choices constantly about how sensibly we wish to live to maintain good health. We are free to ignore such advice and may eventually pay the price, consciously or unconsciously. Since excessive Vata implies nervous tension or excitability, another recommendation was to take warm baths for relaxation in the morning. This struck me as unusual, since I rarely took relaxing baths, and if I had in the past, they would always be in the evening. It seemed odd at first, but the process turned out to be a pleasant one.

There were many other recommendations that included some adjustments in diet, foods to emphasize and some to avoid. A herbal preparation was also prescribed, to be taken for two months. I was not actively troubled by any specific physical or mental symptoms at the time of this examination. It was primarily an evaluation to use for

health maintenance and prevention. The elimination of coffee and alcohol was also recommended. The number of recommendations were more than I felt ready to follow in
their entirety. Those that I was able and willing to do, however, I did find useful, and
clearly not harmful. The program of action included several self-massage techniques
using warm sesame oil. These are relaxing and pleasant. I was advised to include meditation practice twice a day for twenty minutes. Since I had been practicing meditation
for almost a year, I was already carrying out this recommendation. There have been
scientific studies of meditation over the past twenty years, with sufficient evidence that
it is an effective stress reduction procedure. Although my blood pressure had always
been normal, usually averaging about 120/80, I did find that several months of practicing meditation lowered my blood pressure to about 105/65, accompanied by a slower
pulse rate.

Diet, exercise, daily routine, and seasonal routine are the four most common means
to promote and maintain balance in Ayurvedic medical care. These are mainly for prevention and not sufficient for treating diseases. A more complete medical regimen
might include other methods, such as additional herbal preparations, music therapy,
aromatherapy, and several other procedures that require specialized training for proper
administration, such as *panchakarma therapy*, which is a program of five ("pancha"
means five) cleansings. The classic method includes emetics, purgatives, and enemas.

Some forms of Panchakarma use an intensive series of oil massages, emetics, herbal
enemas, sweat treatments, and nasal inhalations, administered over a period of at least
several days. When I attended an annual meeting of the American Association of Ayurvedic Medicine in 1990, I met a psychiatrist from a Midwestern state who had undergone a week of panchakarma. He told me that it was the most profound experience of
relaxation he had ever had. One oil massage is particularly remarkable, called *Shi-
rodhara*, in which warm herbalized sesame oil is dripped in a stream onto the forehead
for more than an hour. This produces a state of profound relaxation of the nervous system. This is a method to balance Prana Vata, a subdosha that exerts major control over
the brain. The psychiatrist told me that his cholesterol level had been three hundred
milligrams percent when he went for the treatment. A week later it had dropped to one
hundred and fifty. The program of treatment was residential in his case, and this included eating only vegetarian food, which also would have had an effect on his cholesterol level. Panchakarma is also used as a health maintenance practice that can be
undertaken two or three times a year.

Dr. Robert Svoboda has also written a small, well-written booklet, *The Hidden
Secret of Ayurveda* (Svoboda, 1980). Dr. Svoboda states that the first axiom in Ayurveda is that "everything that exists in the external universe has its counterpart in the internal universe of the human body." This is the law of the macrocosm, the large world,
existing in or paralleling the microcosm, the small world. The same principle had been
stated by the medieval alchemists of Europe who said: As above, so below, referring to
the Cosmos and the human being.

The second axiom mentioned by Dr. Svoboda is that "Air, fire, and Water are the
three principles most fundamental to life." These match the three doshas already
described. Disease is disharmony of the three, usually due to an increase in one or more

of them. External elements are significant influences, including the seasons themselves and the passage of time. The time of the year and the time of life both affect the internal systems of the body. This is expressed in a third axiom by Dr. Svoboda: "Like increases like." Older age is considered a period for a drying tendency, which is one characteristic of Vata. Therefore, Vata problems can and often do occur in older age.

The place of diet or nutrition is central to Ayurvedic thinking, not only for treatment but especially for prevention of illness. A major emphasis on taste is a distinctive aspect of Ayurveda, more than in most other health and healing systems throughout the world. Six different tastes are described: sweet, sour, salty, pungent, bitter, and astringent. It has been observed that certain tastes either aggravate or pacify different doshas. For example, persons who are predominantly Vata should avoid bitter, pungent and astringent foods in excess, since they increase Air energy and therefore cause gas in the body. Substances containing sweet, sour and salty tastes are good for people with Vata constitutions.

The term, sweet, does not only mean the usual sweetness of sugar, which is a pure form of sweetness, but also includes complex carbohydrates. Dairy, meat, and oils are classified as primarily sweet. The selection of foods by tastes as defined by the Ayurvedic system was developed long before any knowledge of protein, fat and carbohydrate existed, and yet the system appears to work out correctly in relation to a balanced diet. What is good or bad as a food depends on how it affects a particular person.

There is a paradox present in Ayurveda. It can appear simple and unsophisticated in some respects, without the specific drugs of modern medicine. Simultaneously it can be powerful in its effects on the entire mind/body/spirit unity of the person. It does not have to replace or be a substitute for modern medicine, but can be used with it. Several people with advanced cancer are reported (Chopra, 1989) to have obtained better results than had been predicted or expected, when they entered a program that included Ayurvedic methods.

Both Western healers and Ayurvedic physicians emphasize that mental attitude is essential to the healing process. Mental attitude includes consciousness and awareness more than intellectual knowledge. It blends a deep spiritual viewpoint that has been so strikingly absent in Western medicine for the past three hundred years, and especially in the past one hundred years.

There are indications that Ayurveda might become an important health-care system for some developing countries. This could equally become true for industrialized countries, whose citizens are increasingly suffering from chronic diseases, for which Ayurveda can contribute relief and possible cure. It is also a significant system for preventive medicine.

The three systems of healing of China, Japan, and India that have been described all have included the existence and application of a form of energy—Ch'i, Ki, or Prana—that is not readily measurable by Western scientific equipment. For a true meeting of Eastern and Western systems of healing, it may ultimately require new models for research. Meanwhile there are other health-enhancement techniques, also used for healing illness, that use Eastern energy concepts, in the West.

III

Non-Medical Healing:
Eastern and Western

12

Healing Energies

The Eastern traditions of healing have described Ch'i (Qi), Ki, and Prana for many centuries. This subtle energy has been used or mobilized in healing, such as in acupuncture, pulse diagnosis and herbal medicine. Nonetheless Western scientists remain not only skeptical but at times even emotionally irritated by such ideas. There are a few Western scientists and writers who are sympathetic and accepting of the possibility that prana does exist. Fritjof Capra, a quantum physicist, has given support to Eastern views paralleling some findings in post-Einsteinian quantum physics.

In *The Tao of Physics* (Capra, 1975) and *The Turning Point* (Capra, 1982) he proposes that Eastern ways of thinking can contribute to new viewpoints that are evolving in Western society, called paradigm shifts and cultural transformations. The title of *The Turning Point* was taken from the ancient Chinese classic, *The I Ching*. It has been a book for guidance and advice over the millenia. It is composed of sixty-four hexagrams, or six-line passages. Number twenty-four is translated as "Return" or The Turning Point. As described by Richard Wilhelm (Wilhelm, 1967, p.97):

> After a time of decay comes the turning point. The powerful light that has been banished returns. There is movement, but it is not brought about by force. . . The movement is natural, arising spontaneously. For this reason the transformation of the old becomes easy. The old is discarded and the new is introduced. Both measures accord with the time, therefore no harm results.

Capra devotes almost a fourth of *The Turning Point* to health philosophy, conventional and holistic. In *The Tao of Physics* he describes similarities between Eastern philosophy and Western science.

There have always been certain individuals who have had an unusual gift for being able to place their hands on a sick person and produce or mobilize a healing response.

This "laying on of hands" is an ancient tradition, described in the Bible and usually associated with religious or spiritual teachings and practices. Usually, it is called spiritual or psychic healing. It has occurred outside mainstream, secular medicine and science.

In recent decades scientific researchers have measured and documented this kind of healing. Some practitioners of hands-on healing have defined themselves explicitly as following a spiritual or religious orientation. Others have defined themselves as secular healers.

In the 1960s Dr. Bernard Grad of McGill University in Montreal, Canada conducted careful scientific studies of a former Hungarian cavalry officer, Colonel Oscar Estabany. While in the Hungarian cavalry Colonel Estabany discovered his ability to heal horses through his use of laying-on-of-hands. Dr. Grad studied the effects of Estabany's hands on laboratory animals and plants. Several carefully designed research experiments showed that Estabany produced positive results that were statistically significant when he did hands-on healing of mice who had thyroid disease produced through diet and medication. Another experiment on wound-healing in mice also showed a significantly faster rate of healing when exposed to Estabany's hands. Dr. Grad also studied the effect Colonel Estabany had on water used to germinate seeds. The treated seeds grew more vigorously than seeds watered without Estabany's influence.

Richard Gerber, M. D. in *Vibrational Medicine* (Gerber, 1988) describes these experiments in detail. Dr. Gerber's book is an extensive study of "subtle energies," from both a scientific and spiritual viewpoint. Dr. Gerber refers to Estabany's activities as examples of "psychic healing." Simultaneously he frequently refers to the subtle energy as a form of electromagnetic phenomenon. It is not easy to discuss these kinds of processes within the standard categories of present-day science and knowledge.

In 1969 I heard a talk by Dr. Justa Smith, a biochemist and enzymologist who also had studied Colonel Estabany's abilities. Dr. Smith, a professor at Rosary Hill College in Buffalo, New York and director of their Human Dimensions Institute, had heard Dr. Grad report on his research with Estabany. She proposed a research project with the use of digestive enzymes, such as pancreatic trypsin. She had previously studied the effects of high magnetic fields on trypsin, and found that they accelerated the rate of enzyme activity. She then had Estabany apply his skills to test-tubes of enzyme solutions, and found that he had the same effect as the high magnetic fields.

Since healing is an activity for distressed or ill people, Dr. Smith proposed to study Estabany's impact on injured enzymes. By exposing enzymes to ultra-violet radiation, the biological activity of the enzymes was impaired. After Estabany "healed" the injured enzymes, they recovered their normal reactivity, and with further treatment became even more active. Dr. Smith presented a summary of these experiments at the 1972 Dimensions of Healing Symposium held at Stanford University and the University of California in Los Angeles. The presentation is part of a volume prepared by the Academy of Parapsychology and Medicine in 1972.

Dr. Justa Smith also studied a well-known spiritual healer, Olga Worrall, who had the ability to influence biochemical reactions. She and her husband, Ambrose Worrall, an engineer, had conducted healing services in a Methodist church in Baltimore, Maryland for several decades until their death. Dr. Gerber in *Vibrational Medicine* raises the question whether one could train ordinary people to be healers, or "are healers merely an elite group of humans in our society who possess a rare gift at birth?" The answer is a yes; one can train individuals in the health-care professions or interested laypersons to do healing on others.

Therapeutic Touch: Therapeutic Touch is a present-day example of a hands-on healing technique that Dr. Dolores Krieger developed. Dr. Krieger is a professor of nursing at New York University, and an R.N. She had become familiar with Dr. Grad's studies of several healers, including Colonel Estabany. Dr. Krieger had been a member of a team that studied Colonel Estabany in 1971. This research project involved human subjects who were ill and were given laying-on-of-hands treatment by Estabany. The hemoglobin levels of patients were measured and also a control group who did not receive any treatment. There were measurable increases in hemoglobin in the treated group. Another member of the research team was Dora Kunz, a clairvoyant. She had experience in the use of using the hands to heal as well as having the ability to "see auras." Aura is the term for a transparent light effect that surrounds the body but is not usually measurable nor can be photographed. For centuries there have been individuals who have been able to detect these illuminations, though Western scientists have not agreed about their actual existence. These kinds of phenomena are often called "para-normal" and are difficult to prove. Despite this, some childen and a few of the normal adult population can report such sights.

Dora Kunz gave Dr. Krieger instruction in methods of performing the laying on of hands for healing. Later Dr. Krieger developed a course to teach other nurses the art or technique that she eventually called Therapeutic Touch. She found that the more she used it, the more effective were the results. She could increase the speed of recovery of some hospitalized patients. She could observe her students and concluded that individuals who were not naturally psychic or spiritual healers could be taught to do such healing.

Her first book, *The Therapeutic Touch: How to Use Your Hands to Help and Heal* was published in 1979 (Krieger, 1979). The application of Therapeutic Touch to premature babies in one hospital was dramatic in its positive effects. It was also useful in Emergency Room care.

In 1971 a provocative book, *Psychic Discoveries behind the Iron Curtain* was published. I heard one of the authors, Sheila Ostrander, speak at the *Beyond the Senses* conference of the American Academy of Psychotherapists in 1972. She summarized some of the book by saying that the Russians were exploring ways to use psychic skills and phenomena for practical purposes, while at the same time the United States was still debating whether there really was such a phenomenon.

My wife's experiences in Russia confirm these comments. She had participated in the First International Free-Breathers Conference in Moscow, Russia in June of 1991. She was impressed by the advanced development of energy-work used by some of the healers at the conference. She personally experienced a Russian doctor's energy healing of her sore and mildly inflamed knees.

When she was eleven, she had a sledding accident that caused a dislocation of her left knee-cap. This was followed by recurrent dislocations. About twenty years ago she underwent orthopedic surgery to stabilize the knee joint. Since then there has been some restriction of movement in the left leg in bending. When overly stressed physically, pain and swelling often occurs. This would often require one or two weeks of careful pampering to obtain satisfactory relief. The uninjured knee at times would also be sore if excessive strain had occurred.

While staying on the ninth floor of a Moscow hotel for the ten days of the conference, the electricity in that part of the city was not always working. Therefore, she had to walk up and down the stairs several times a day. This led to pain and swelling in both knees. One of the Russian hosts became aware of her physical problem and said, "We have many healers in our group. I will bring one of them to you."

At eleven in the evening, after the evening conference activities finished, Sasha appeared with the host who had made the offer. Sasha was a small, gentle, alert doctor in his midthirties. My wife's journal of her trip described the experience with the comment, "He asked me all about my knees and what had been my feelings at that time [of the surgery] in my life. [There was no translator present and his English was modest at best]."

What came out from the questioning was the story of what had happened after surgery on the left knee. The surgeon had totally discounted her complaint of pain in the knee while it was in a leg cast. When the cast was finally removed, the knee area was markedly swollen and there was evidence that there had been infection post-operatively, as revealed by enlarged suture marks, which had already healed. Later she learned that this particular surgeon had a reputation of having too many patients develop post-operative infections. Sasha asked her if she could forgive and try to love the surgeon. She hadn't fully realized how much resentment and anger were still present inside her. She further reported in her journal:

> He [Sasha] did not touch me other than the handshake of introduction. He then asked me to write my full name on a piece of paper for him, and asked me to lie down on the bed, eyes closed, and concentrate on love and forgiveness, especially for myself and Dr. C [the orthopedic surgeon]. Sasha then sat on the floor across the room in lotus position, leaning against a big suitcase.
>
> Within a minute or two, I felt swirls of energy in my head, more powerful than any Reiki treatment I've ever experienced [She has ten years of familiarity with Reiki]. It then traveled down each arm. I continued to concentrate on loving and forgiving myself and my doctor, while the swirling energies started again in my head and this time slowly swirled down each leg. After about fifteen minutes he got up, came over, held my hand, and looked very deeply into my eyes. My tears started to roll. He said that since the problems were so old (about twenty years) it would need two to three more sessions. He said he normally only needs to do one [treatment].

She woke up the next morning with all the swelling gone from the right knee and considerably less swelling in the left knee [the one operated on], and free of all pain. She wrote, "This is amazing as I have a twenty-year pattern of needing 1 to 2 weeks of real pampering to heal an inflamed knee." By evening the swelling had eased even more, despite more stair-climbing, when the electricity was off, and the elevators couldn't operate. Sasha gave her a second healing session late in the evening of this second day. She wrote what happened:

> It was different from last night. This time the energy swirled all through my body at the same time, not inch by inch. After about ten minutes, Sasha got up from the floor on the other side of the room, and knelt by my bed, and held my right hand in his, tightly. I have never felt such current [of energy]. As I was wondering how he could also hold my right foot in his hand so firmly, I realized that he wasn't doing this physically. He stroked my hand for a minute, smiled, and told me to thank God, thank myself, and have a good sleep.

On the third day Sasha came to give a third healing session in the evening. Sasha is a physician who works in a hospital. He has also had training in Reiki and uses ancient Russian healing methods. Again, from Jean's journal:

> His healing energy is so powerful, it is hard to believe. Tonight's session was quite different from the previous two. I felt the energy swirling down through my head to feet, then head, shoulders, and down each arm, back to my knees and ankles. Then came the shocker—it zinged and ricocheted all through my torso—hard to describe. [Sasha] has the petiteness of Sammy Davis Jr., a ready smile, and is obviously a compassionate, noninvasive person.

Sasha came a fourth night. She went to his room for the final session. "He doesn't know if this session will complete my process [it did]. I do know my knees haven't felt this good for years. He sat on the far side, as usual. The energy came and grew as in previous nights." For the rest of the trip to Russia her knees caused no pain, swelling or other problems, despite more walking and climbing.

In December of 1991 my wife and I had a visit from a young Russian woman who is a Physician's Assistant. She had been at the Moscow conference. She conducts a healing practice in a government clinic, where she also uses Reiki healing combined with energy-healing. I was able to watch a video recording of her conducting a healing session on an American in northern Maine, that she had carried out several days earlier. She did not touch him physically but moved her arms and hands up and down his body, several inches away from the body while he was standing. This was followed by a standard Reiki [Reiki Alliance] treatment while he was lying down. It is difficult in words to describe what occurs, since it is visually vivid.

The Russians, faced with a great deal of limited technology in medicine, find it useful to apply energy healing methods. They clearly are less skeptical or negative about it. Even before present-day technological advances, Russia has had a tradition for centuries of energy healing.

Reiki: Since the opening of contact between the West and Japan in the 1860s, there has been a constant flow back and forth of ideas and cultural elements to each other. As mentioned earlier George Ohsawa and Macrobiotics began in Japan but did not become a central part of its healing and medical practices. It was brought to Europe and the United States, and only lately has it been imported back to Japan on a small scale.

The story of Reiki and its travels has a somewhat similar history, although it has not yet returned to where it originated, in Japan, to any significant degree. Reiki is a system that is based on the principles of Ki, or universal life energy. The Ki is passed through a Reiki practitioner to a person seeking healing energy. The founder of Reiki was a Japanese Christian educator, Dr. Mikao Usui. Dr. Usui taught in a Christian school in Kyoto in the late nineteenth century.

When confronted by some of his students to explain how Jesus performed the healing miracles reported in the New Testament, Dr. Usui realized he could not give satisfactory answers. This impelled him to depart for the United States and study in a theological seminary in Chicago, Illinois for several years, where he also earned a doctorate in theology. He did not find satisfaction in his quest for answers. He returned to Japan and continued his search.

He spent several more years in a Zen Buddhist monastery studying traditional Zen healing methods. This led him to study Chinese texts, and finally to learn Sanskrit in order to study early Indian texts, and some Tibetan writings. Finally, he decided to undertake an extended fast and meditation for twenty-one days on the top of Mt. Kuriyama, a traditional holy site, near Kyoto. After the twenty-one days passed, he experienced an unusual episode of enlightenment that was both an intense mystical experience and the revelation of a set of symbols to use for healing.

Growing out of this experience, he developed Reiki as a system of healing, after he discovered that he had developed effective healing powers. He carried out healing at first in the worst slums of a city, but later developed a clinic. There he trained others and carried out healing on large numbers of people. His closest collaborator, whom he had taught, was Dr. Chijiro Hayashi, a Reserve Naval Officer. Dr. Hayashi continued to run a private clinic in Tokyo after Dr. Usui died sometime after World War I. Eventually about twenty Reiki clinics were established before World War II. Dr. Usui had appointed Dr. Hayashi as Grand Reiki Master to carry on the Reiki tradition. Dr. Hayashi practiced Reiki for at least twenty years until 1941. He died shortly before the beginning of World War II.

Before he died, Dr. Hayashi appointed as Reiki Grand Master, in an unusual action, a woman and a non-Japanese citizen, Hawayo Takata of Hawaii. Hawayo Takata was born in 1900 on the island of Kauai to parents who had emigrated from Japan five years earlier. As a young woman she had become a housekeeper for a large plantation estate owner, where she worked for twenty-four years. She married the plantation company bookkeeper, Saichi Takata, had two daughters, and became a widow when her husband died at thirty-four. Five years later in 1935 she found herself emotionally drained and physically ill. She had been advised to have abdominal surgery. Then a sister died while her parents were spending a year at the family home in Yamaguchi, Japan, after being away forty years. Mrs. Takata went to Japan to take her husband's ashes back to his ancestral home, inform her parents of the death of the sister, and undergo medical and surgical treatment herself for a tumor, gallstones, and appendicitis. At the last moment before surgery she decided to postpone it.

She had been referred by a doctor to the Reiki clinic run by Dr. Hayashi and his sixteen associates. She experienced so much relief that she continued receiving Reiki sessions until she felt markedly improved. She then asked to be allowed to learn Reiki herself. Despite the prevailing restrictions at the time not to allow it outside Japan, and the fact that Mrs. Takata was a woman, she was given permission. After a year of training and practice she was admitted to the more advanced form of Reiki, the Second Degree, or Practitioner's Level.

She returned to Hawaii in the summer of 1937. A few weeks later Dr. Hayashi visited Hawaii and spent six months there, to help establish Reiki there. Before he returned to Japan he chose Mrs. Takata to be a Reiki Master. She was then qualified to teach and initiate students, and be a practitioner. She established a center on the island of Hawaii at Hilo. She became very popular, teaching Reiki throughout the islands and visiting villages to give Reiki "treatments" or sessions.

Mrs. Takata returned to Japan for a visit to Dr. Hayashi shortly before his death. He then appointed her to be his successor as Reiki Grand Master. Before assuming the mantle and responsibilities in Japan, she decided first to return home to Hawaii for awhile, to put her affairs in order and to complete the raising of her children. Then she would return to Japan. When World War II began shortly afterward, all communication was cut off for more than the four years of the war. By the time Mrs. Takata was able to return to Japan, almost all signs of Reiki activity had disappeared, and there were no practitioners remaining. She then decided to return to Hawaii and spread the Reiki message and conduct training from her center in Hawaii. She continued her work there for the next thirty years until her death in 1980.

In 1973, as described by Helen Haberly in *Hawayo Takata's Story* (Haberly, 1990), "[Takata] was invited to teach a large group on an island off the coast of Washington state, and this was the start of seven very busy years." Previously most of her work in Hawaii had been with the Japanese communities of Hawaii. At this point she began to travel throughout the United States and Canada.

The demands for teaching became so great that she trained some of her students to be initiated as Reiki Masters in the last few years of her life. A gathering of twenty-one American Reiki Masters occurred in 1980 to form an organization. Mrs. Takata's granddaughter, Phyllis Lee Furamoto was appointed by her to be her successor. Earlier in 1976 Mrs. Takata did visit Japan and gave First Degree, or basic Reiki, training to three hundred Japanese people, and Second Degree, or Advanced Reiki, to fifteen Japanese.

Since her death two organizations of Reiki practitioners have been established. One is the Reiki Alliance, with Phyllis Furamoto as Reiki Grand Master. She has continued to teach in Germany and in the United States, also in other parts of the world. The other Reiki organization is the Radiance Technique Association International (formerly the American International Reiki Association, Inc.) founded by Dr. Barbara Weber Ray of Atlanta, Georgia. Dr. Ray is one of the twenty-one Americans trained by Mrs. Takata to carry on the Reiki tradition. Both Barbara Ray and Phyllis Furamoto are considered Reiki Grand Master by their respective organizations, carrying on the tradition of Reiki healing established by Mikao Usui.

There are Reiki practitioners throughout all parts of the United States, Canada, Germany and the Soviet Union. One estimate of people trained in Reiki in the United States is one hundred thousand. There are physicians, nurses, chiropractors, and massage therapists who have trained in Reiki. There are also many laypersons who can use it for themselves, their family and friends, their pets and their houseplants.

It is appropriate to ask: exactly what is Reiki? It is a process in which the Reiki practitioner places her hands very gently on the fully clothed body of a person, in a variety of established places on the head, chest, abdomen, and back for one or more minutes in each position. In addition areas of the body where there is pain or other physical symptoms or signs also may receive Reiki treatment through the hands of the practitioner. The purpose is to affect the body, mind or spirit of the recipient to mobilize whatever healing is sought. The practitioner is not defined as the one who is performing the healing. He is only a conduit for the universal energy, or Ki, or whatever term one might choose to call it. The process also can be carried out with the hands just slightly off the surface of the body, as in some forms of Polarity Therapy.

In both First Degree and Second Degree training, which each takes place over a two day period, there is an attunement, or initiation procedure, by the Reiki Master. This is intended to open the trainee more fully to the flow of Ki. This attunement endows the trainee with a permanent access to Ki, greater than had been possible before the initiations. The Second Degree training with further attunements and instructions allows for a more powerful effect by the practitioner. It also includes additional training to carry out mental/psychological healing, and healing at a distance, or absentee healing. None of this is contrary to nor antagonistic to any conventional medical or surgical treatment methods.

My personal experience with Reiki supports this. I enrolled in a First Degree Reiki Workshop in 1986 with the Reverend David Jarrell, a Reiki Master who was one of the twenty-one Americans trained by Hawayo Takata. It happened to be a few days after I underwent a radioactive scan of my thyroid because of suspicion of a thyroid tumor (which was there). This also coincided with an attack of neck pain due to osteoarthritis for which I had consulted a family physician. A fortunate result of the visit to him led to the radioactive scan. Although the neck pain had not been severe, the physical requirements of the scan demanded that I lie down on the x-ray table with my head bent back as far as possible, in a hyperextended position. This produced excruciating pain for the eight minutes necessary to hold absolutely still, while the scan was completed. At one point I was not sure I could complete the procedure because of the severity of the pain.

Three days later I was asked to lie face down on a massage table as part of the first day of the Reiki training. My neck was still moderately painful. The seven other trainees and the Reiki Master applied Reiki to me. This was not only for training practice for the group, but also was a healing session to give me some relief for my still aching and painful neck.

The next day I again received a session on the table, but by then I had no discomfort or pain in my neck at all. Nothing like it has recurred in the following six years. I admit this is not a scientific report or study. It is also true, as my family physician pointed out, that acute attacks can be self-limiting in a few weeks. Nonetheless, I was profoundly delighted to experience such total relief. I had not been taking any pain medicine during the several days of the Reiki training. I have since heard many other reports of the healing value of Reiki from others, including the experience of other Reiki practitioners.

I have more recently undertaken Second Degree Reiki training with another Reiki Master, the Reverend John Harvey Gray. John Gray was in the first group of Americans who received training from Mrs. Takata. Since then he has conducted approximately four hundred training workshops throughout the United States, with a total of about three thousand students. Although I cannot speak from any extensive experience in conducting Reiki sessions on individuals, it is clear to me that it never does any harm, and can be useful both for health maintenance and for enhancing healing of any kind.

Bodo Baginski and Shalila Sharamon, both Reiki practitioners, describe some effects Reiki can have in *Reiki: Universal Life Energy* (Baginski & Sharamon, 1988):

> Reiki supports the body's natural ability to heal itself ;
> Reiki vitalizes both body and soul ;
> Reiki reestablishes spiritual equilibrium and mental well-being ;
> Reiki functions on all levels, whether mental or
>   spiritual, bodily or emotional ;
> Reiki balances the body's energies ;
> Reiki loosens up blocked energy and promotes a state of total relaxation ;
> Reiki cleanses the body of poisons ;
> Reiki adjusts itself according to the needs of the recipient ;
> Reiki works with animals and plants ; and
> Reiki is an extremely pleasant, holistic method of healing.

Two or more practitioners can work together, or even a group can, as in my first experience. A Reiki session usually lasts twenty minutes, and on rare occasion one or more hours. Although the Radiance Technique International Association conducts research as one of its several activities, Reiki remains, like many other nonconventional healing aids, scientifically unproven, but frequently helpful.

Reiki promotes healing through methods that are rooted in a spiritual tradition. Psychological and physical processes are not directly involved. The recipient is asked only to lie comfortably on a mat or table usually, although Reiki can be given to anyone wherever they are sitting or lying down. There are no specific instructions given about breathing.

Polarity Therapy: The originators of osteopathy, chiropractic, and homeopathy— Still, Palmer, and Hahnemann—all believed in an intrinsic energy that flows within the bodymind and is also the expression of a broader universal energy, as defined in Chinese and Indian healing as Ch'i(Qi) or Prana. Based on these ideas of energy flow and its blockage, Dr. Randolph Stone created a blend of Eastern and Western systems of healing, which he called Polarity Therapy.

Dr. Stone represents a good example of the meeting of East and West within one person. He was born in Austria in 1890 and came to the United States in 1903. Later he studied osteopathy, chiropractic, and naturopathy in the United States. He also spent several years in India where he learned about Ayurveda. He practiced for many years in Chicago, Illinois, but also traveled extensively throughout the world, moved to India for several years, and then returned to the United States. He retired to India when he was eighty-one and lived there for another ten years until his death at ninety-one in 1981.

His first book that expressed his views on healing was *The New Energy Concept of the Healing Art* in 1948. A later version was titled *Energy: The Vital Polarity in the Healing Art* (Stone, date unknown). He called his entire approach to health and healing Polarity Therapy. He believed that there was an energy flow in and between people that was electromagnetic in character. Positive and negative poles existed in every cell of the body as well as a general polarity of the entire body. In Dr. Stone's opinion, the head has a positive charge and the feet a negative one.

He also used ideas identical with Ayurveda, such as his reference to five elements— ether, air, fire, water, and earth—all created from the energetic movements in the body. He developed techniques for balancing the energies of the body through touch, by placing the hands in specific parts of the body that were considered positive and negative. Occasionally firmer pressure was used. In addition Dr. Stone designed stretching techniques to be applied by the therapists, and stretching exercises to be done by the patient.

Dr. Stone developed other activities besides the energy balancing work in Polarity Therapy. He recommended attention to proper diet and nutrition, recommended a vegetarian diet, and proper exercise. He developed a system of exercises he called *Polarity Yoga*. He also believed in adequate intestinal care, partly derived from Ayurveda and from European traditions. He also recommended a process called "liver flush" for stimulating the liver and gall-bladder. The purpose was not only to release bile but presumably to discharge "wastes and toxins." There is no question that the ingestion of olive oil and citric juices will stimulate the gall-bladder vigorously. I am familiar with one example of this in a slightly modified form.

When one of my daughters was sixteen, a friend of the family told her about the liver flush. I am not at all clear why the recommendation was given. Nonetheless, my daughter was adventuresome enough to carry out the procedure. She drank several ounces of olive oil, and ate several grapefruit. She then lay down on the bed on her right side, and rested for several hours. When "Nature took its course" with the gall-bladder's reaction to the high fat ingestion, and whatever specific effect the grapefruit produced, she noticed that she had passed several green marble-like objects, which may well have been very early stages of gallstones. I do not recommend anyone do this by themselves, without medical advice or professional guidance of some type.

Polarity Therapy incorporates the use of the chakra system as found in Ayurveda. Some of the balancing includes techniques that are considered a form of chakra balancing. Sometimes the therapist may not touch the body of the person receiving treatment, but move the hands along the body an inch or two away from the body. This is consistent with a viewpoint that an energy field exists around the body that is not identical with pure physical energy, such as heat and cold.

There is an American Polarity Therapy Association with several hundred members, and a training program to become a Polarity Therapist. A similar organization exists in England, with registered practitioners and a three-year training program.

There are no specific breathing techniques usually accompanying most energy healing approaches. It is relevant, however, that the Greek, Hebrew, and Arabic words for Spirit are the same ones used for "breath." To breathe in is to inspire, and inspiration refers not only to breath, but to an emotional or spiritual experience.

13

Breathwork

Since ancient times there has existed a belief that the mind and spirit have a connection to the breath. Both the Hebrew, *ruach*, and the Greek, *pneuma,* are words for Spirit. They also mean "breath." In Genesis in the Old Testament God is described as making man from the clay of the earth and bringing life to him by breathing into him. Mouth-to-mouth resuscitation, through breathing into the recipient mechanically, can revive a person who has stopped breathing and would otherwise have died. The conventional medical definition of a live newborn requires that the infant has taken its first breath. In some spiritual traditions it is believed that the soul enters the body at the time of the first breath. This is the moment that is used by professional astrologers to calculate an exact chart, or *horoscope.*

We can go without food for more than a month. We can go without water for several days, but we cannot go without air for more than a few minutes. Breath is Life. It is not coincidental that the word, inspiration, means "to breathe air in" or inhalation, and has the meaning of "stimulation of the mind or emotions to a high level of feeling or activity." The American Heritage dictionary also defines inspiration as "Divine guidance or influence exerted directly upon the mind and soul of man." Similarly the word, expiration, means "the act of breathing out" and "to die, to come to a close or end."

In the practice of Yoga, there is an extensive system of breathing techniques, called *Pranayama*. The purpose is to control or direct the breath to restore and maintain health and simultaneously develop a higher state of spiritual evolution or consciousness. In the West Yoga, particularly Hatha Yoga, is used to create relaxation and improve general health. In the Hindu tradition pranayama is intended to produce higher states of consciousness through a variety of breathing techniques. There is no complete separation of mind and body, so that mental balance is as much a factor in creating physical health as physical activity by itself. The breath is the connection between the mind and the body. Breathing is the only physiological process in the body that is under both voluntary and involuntary control.

Without any conscious attention, the body will carry out breathing automatically. Conscious attention by the mind can change the breathing rate and depth in either direction. There are also powerful unconscious factors that can change the depth or quality of breathing. Different emotions affect breathing both acutely and chronically. Fear restricts or even stops breathing momentarily. A reaction of amazement can produce a gasp. Anger can be accompanied by an agitated type of breathing. Relief may produce a sigh. It is not merely a verbal expression when someone says, "I barely have time to breathe." Working under a sense of pressure restricts the movement of the chest muscles that help breathing. The respiratory movements can become restricted. A large percent of the population has restricted breathing, but are not aware of it because it has become so chronic and unconscious.

I have never had any physical problems related to breathing. Up to the age of forty-three I had never paid any attention to how I breathed. The automatic process of my body operated without my giving it any thought. In 1968 I attended a brief workshop in San Francisco, California given by Magda Proskauer, a physiotherapist who had incorporated psychological considerations into her work. She had developed a series of exercises that increased self-awareness about one's breathing. She pointed out that noticing how one breathes can help correct irregularities in breathing. This in turn can lead to a calmer state emotionally and mentally. Three years later I began to study and undertake a form of body-oriented psychotherapy called Bioenergetic Analysis, developed by Alexander Lowen, M. D. One of its central principles and actions is the role of breathing in emotional states and their resolution. My breathing and its restrictions were a major focus, besides working with other muscular restrictions and understanding more about my personality.

As a person breathes more deeply, deep emotions may arise, including sobbing, laughing, and sometimes increased anxiety on its way toward discharge. Especially in men, the chest muscles that are part of the breathing mechanism can become so constricted and tight that it is easy to compare them to rusty barrel staves that allow only a small amount of movement. This may be far less than what the lungs can take in. Physical rigidity and emotional rigidity are two forms of the same state of being.

There is a special type of breathing process that is not a therapy, but has many benefits for those who learn and practice it, a special form of conscious breathing known as *Rebirthing*. In the early 1970s in California, Leonard Orr developed a process that he initially called Rebirthing but later called simply *Conscious Breathing* (Orr & Ray, 1977). Conscious Connected Breathing or Circular Breathing are alternate terms for this process. In Russia it is called *Free Breathing*. Leonard Orr was an active participant in the Human Potential Movement in California in the late 1960s and 1970s. At first he had participants go through a process in warm water in a hot tub, with a snorkel, lying face down in the water. The purpose was to evoke memories, images, and sensations of the original birth experience. As he experimented with hundreds of participants, he eventually found that a "dry birth" process was equally effective, and simpler to conduct. Gradually he developed a technique that not only allowed for the release of emotional conflicts relating to birth, or birth trauma, but also early memories and experiences in the first four or five years of life surfaced, as well as more recent emotional conflicts.

One of Leonard Orr's colleagues in the development of this process is Sondra Ray. She has written several books that elaborate on rebirthing (Ray, 1983) and other aspects of personal growth, which she has called *Loving Relationships Training*, or LRT. Leonard Orr created a center in California where he teaches rebirthing for those who wish to become professional rebirthers. He has conducted workshops in Poland and Russia, other parts of Europe and throughout the United States. Many of his students have also developed programs for teaching trainees, and conducting individual and group rebirthing sessions for tens of thousand of citizens. There are more than one thousand rebirthers in the United States and several hundred in other countries, including Russia.

In 1972 I met a woman in New York City, Elizabeth Feher, who had independently developed her own form of rebirthing. She was a group therapist who had her patients go through an experience that was designed to simulate their original physical birth. She used a thin pad, about thirty feet long, on the floor of her loft office. The person undergoing this process would lie down on their back with their knees bent. Elizabeth Feher would then have the person put their hands up and press against hers. The person was asked to take three slow, deep breaths, and then "skootch" along the pad with the help of an assistant. The person was free to go along the pad as far as they felt the need and then pivot around and come back to the beginning. If they needed more time and distance, they could repeat the journey as much as needed. After they finished, they were accompanied by two assistants to the bathroom, left alone to empty the bladder, and then return on their own. Then they were given crackers and milk and held in someone's arms. It was a combination of reliving birth and early childhood. I participated in this four times.

Mrs. Feher knew absolutely nothing about my personal history except that I was a psychiatrist. Her comment to me after the several rebirthings I undertook was, "You have been rushed a lot." I laughed with the shock of recognition that her statement was so true. Not only was I the third of three children, without any history of obstetrical difficulty, but it also was true that from age four to twenty-nine, I had experienced what I could call "rushing" in my life, especially educationally, for several reasons.

Mrs. Feher had noticed in the body movements and actions of the many rebirthings she had facilitated that they contained expressions of the original birth experience. In several cases she was able to have the patient obtain information from their mothers about their birth. There were interesting similarities between the rebirthing and the original one. In one case a woman suddenly stopped during her rebirthing, paused for several minutes, and then continued her rebirthing on the long mattress-like pad. Information was obtained later that her mother had been heavily anesthetized during labor, and it had stopped for awhile. I also learned that the patient herself had struggled with an alcohol problem in recent years.

Mrs. Feher had demonstrated her method to a few professionals in England and in the United States. Unfortunately, she died of influenza a year or two after my contact with her, before she could write about her observations. Her daughter, Leslie Feher, also a psychologist, continued the interest in birth psychology by forming an organization to study birth psychology.

One of Sigmund Freud's earliest colleagues, Otto Rank, wrote a book on "The Birth

Trauma" in the 1920s. In it he proposed a theory that the experience of birth can contribute to later emotional problems, and was the primary source of anxiety. The experience and observations of many present-day rebirthers would appear to confirm both Rank and Leonard Orr's ideas about birth trauma. Neither Leonard Orr nor other rebirthers limit the value of rebirthing to birth trauma resolution. Residues of parental disapproval, early pre-verbal and non-verbal upsets are also commonly reexperienced during a breathing session.

In June of 1991 the First Annual Free-Breathers Conference was convened in Moscow, Russia for ten days. I am familiar with what occurred, since my wife, Jean, was one of ten Americans who participated in it as faculty leaders, at the invitation of the founder and coordinator of the International Association for Free Breathing, Sergei Vschsvyatski. Some of the Americans were members of the Rebirthers Association of New England and the rest were rebirthers from other parts of the United States.

Two hundred and thirty-seven enrollees from all parts of the Soviet Union attended, and a few Germans. More than half the enrollees were Soviet physicians. Most of the enrollees were rebirthers who had been trained three years before by Leonard Orr and Sondra Ray in Russia.

Before the Moscow conference, some of the Americans traveled to the Republic of Georgia near the Black Sea. They gave lectures, and also conducted group and individual rebirthings. One Georgian physician who had heard lectures by the group in Georgia had a session of rebirthing. He then decided to attend the Moscow conference, because of his introduction. The Americans spent five days in Georgia in a small city near Tiblisi, the capital. The bus-driver who accompanied the group for the several days became so intrigued by what he observed that he asked for a session. He joined the last group session scheduled for the next day.

This took place the morning the group was to be driven to the airport, on their way to Moscow. After the driver finished his rebirthing session, he was so relaxed and not fully "integrated" that another bus-driver had to be recruited, while the bus-driver became a passenger with the Americans. He was so delighted with his experience that he contributed to the farewell celebration at the airport in characteristic generous Georgian style by treating everyone to a small banquet while they waited for their plane.

Rebirthing usually consists of a session for one to two hours in which the person lies down on a comfortable mat, and simply breathes in a circular manner. Just as the inhalation ends, the exhalation is started without any pause. The exhalation is usually a simple letting-go without any forcing. At the end of exhalation, the breath is immediately inhaled without pause. In regular or yogic breathing there is often a natural pause at the end of exhalation, especially if there has been some deepening of inhalation. In rebirthing this pause is consciously omitted, so that the circular breathing is both at the end of exhalation as well as inhalation; hence the name, *Conscious Connected Breathing*.

For beginners there is often a tendency to force the breathing a little. This frequently leads to some mild symptoms that commonly occur with hyperventilation, such as a tightening of the muscles in the fingers or around the mouth, or some tingling of the hands. The role of the rebirther is to encourage the rebirthee gently to "breathe through it" so that the symptoms will disappear. Many rebirthers will use soft music in the background, both to encourage relaxation and to muffle any distracting sounds that might be heard from outside the room. During the breathing process the senses become much more acute, especially hearing. Usually the rebirthee has the eyes closed.

Breathing may be done through the nose or the mouth, but not usually both. The breathing continues steadily without pause for an extended time. This leads to an altered state of consciousness. The rebirther only speaks occasionally to help the person to keep their focus on their breathing, or to assist if there are any problems, such as the development of hyperventilation symptoms. The key phrase for the rebirthee is "trust the process."

After a period of time, usually at least twenty minutes, but often in the beginning sessions up to forty-five minutes, the rebirthee moves into a state that will vary from person to person. I have observed several dozen rebirthings both in groups and individually, and assisted as a rebirther in some group sessions. Some individuals "bliss out" into a physical state that is striking when observed for the first time. The rebirthee appears to be breathing scarcely at all. Their color is normal but they seem to be in a state of mild suspended animation. Sometimes they may remain in this condition for another half hour or more, and then gradually stir, open their eyes, and finish with their session. They may or may not recall any thoughts or feelings.

Later sessions may be different. More commonly the rebirthee, after the initial period of full deep circular breathing, begins to experience some form of emotional release. It may be experienced quietly with little external signs, or it can become expressive, with crying, sobbing, screaming, shouting, or another type of emotional discharge. They may later report a variety of images or memories, and sometimes an awareness of an answer to a problem that had been present. The process is not intended to be psychotherapy, or physical healing. The rebirther usually does not engage in much verbal interchange. Nonetheless, some rebirthees derive positive results that have psychotherapeutic value, or may experience physical healing.

My first experience of group rebirthing was in 1987 at the Maine Healing Arts Festival. I enrolled in a two-part workshop in rebirthing. There were about twenty in it. We paired up so that one person was to be the rebirther and the other was to be rebirthed. After the first session, we switched in order for everyone to have both experiences. The leader was a psychiatrist who had also conducted individual and group rebirthings for some years as part of his practice. One unusual feature of the sessions was their location outdoors at the edge of a lake. This conference was held at a children's camp shortly after it had closed for the season. The rebirthings took place with the participants spread out along the three sides of the floating dock, typical of children's camps with an enclosed area of water within the three sides. The weather was clear, and comfortable, with blue sky and many pine trees around the lake and on the shore of the camp. Since I had been the rebirther for my partner the first day, I was lying on the dock the next day, with a sleeping bag underneath me for padding.

After I had been breathing steadily for about half an hour, I began to develop the heartiest and strongest belly-laughing that I had ever experienced. This continued for about five minutes or more. I also felt a strong sensation in both my palms that is somewhat difficult to describe. It was extremely pleasurable, and felt like a streaming of energy that was not exactly electrical but was intense. When I opened my eyes, my partner was looking down at me with a beautiful smile. My thought at that moment was, "I have all this wonderful excess energy in my hands, I wish I could use it to heal any-body who might need it." My partner later said that she felt a sensation of heat pouring out of my hands.

The next day the twenty of us who had been in the workshop became rebirthers for as many of the other conference enrollees as wished to participate in a group rebirthing. About sixty people came for the experience. Typical responses occurred, with the majority expressing pleasure at their experience.

There is no evidence there is anything harmful or hurtful in this process, since the rebirthee is totally in control of the process to the extent that they wish to allow the process to unfold. The rebirther is present to be supportive and encouraging, also attend to any needs, such as supplying a kleenex, or wiping tears if necessary. Some rebirthers are professionals, such as nurses, physicians, massage therapists, or spiritual counsel-ors. These rebirthers may include some elements of their usual professional practices intuitively, but this is not really necessary, nor always advisable. The professional may have more to unlearn than the person trained as a rebirther who is a nonprofessional.

The process is humanistic and transpersonal. This means that the relationship between the rebirther and rebirthee is closer to that of equals, and also there are strong spiritual elements involved in the process. As mentioned before, the breath is the link to both body and mind and to "higher consciousness," an element of both the religious and spiritual domain. Some rebirthers refer to the process as a form of "active meditation." Rebirthing is both an art and a science, although there has not been formal research about it, as far as I know.

A frequent but not invariable recommendation by rebirthers for anyone undertaking it is ten rebirthing sessions. Usually, these are at least a week apart, although they can be further apart. Some rebirthers do not require a commitment to the ten sessions, and some do. A person can do their own self-rebirthing whenever they wish. It is easier once they have had a series with a trained rebirther. At first it would be more difficult for a person to allow themselves the depth of letting go, if they were to rebirth themselves. It may strike some as surprising that many people can participate in a group rebirthing and allow themselves emotional release in the presence of others. Sometimes the energy of the group, including whatever sounds are heard, encourages release as much as hinders it. Sometimes a person has a single rebirthing, such as I have described at the Healing Arts Festival, and later decides they wish to pursue it further. On the other hand some people can only engage well in a private session, at least initially.

Among the early students of Leonard Orr were Jim Leonard and Phil Laut, who have written one of the several books on rebirthing (Leonard & Laut, 1983). They have developed their particular form of rebirthing, called *Vivation*. The subtitle of their book, *Rebirthing*, is: *The Science of Enjoying All of Your Life.* They explain in a recent brochure describing Vivation, "It is a highly effective, easy-to-learn self-development technique that enables a person to reconcile and make peace with even the most troub-ling emotions, thereby increasing one's personal effectiveness and peace of mind."

They also state in *Rebirthing* (Leonard & Laut, 1983) that rebirthing "is not therapy, religion, psychology, medicine, hypnosis, or anything to join, and is not a substitute for any of these things."

From my knowledge of individuals who have undertaken a series of rebirthing sessions with my wife, some were able to improve their creativity in writing or musical abilities. Some have found that they could make decisions about career or career changes, or other important decisions in their lives with less conflict. I have called it a "psychic sauna." My wife explains, in an introductory discussion to all her rebirthees, that it is not necessary to examine the contents of the garbage bags on a Saturday morning when putting them out for collection. One merely puts them out without stopping halfway to the curb to examine them. She then points out that the same truth applies to rebirthing. A person may get rid of "mental garbage" without necessarily examining it or figuring out how it got there. Traumas or events that happened in the past cannot be changed, but one can "let go of the charge they hold for you."

Rebirthing as a self-development technique for any interested citizen is part of a larger trend toward self-responsibility and self-improvement. The rebirther is more like a midwife who helps in a natural process than a conventional obstetrician of twenty years ago who was in charge of birth as a medical/surgical procedure. Obviously a well-trained obstetrician is still essential today for any birth that has special problems associated with it, also for those who prefer to have a physician. Similarly, many individuals with complex emotional or mental problems will seek the help of a psychiatrist, psychologist or other mental health professional. Many others are finding that a series of rebirthings can help them resolve some of their life dilemmas.

There are several other forms of breathwork that are available to help in either self-development or as a therapeutic method. Stanislaus Grof, M. D. is a psychiatrist and psychoanalyst who has done much creative exploration in several directions, including psychedelic research. In more recent years he has developed a system called *Holonomic Breathwork* or therapy. His approach includes more intensive sensory bombardment with sound and visual stimuli with circular breathing. There are certifed Holonomic Breath practitioners who have undergone a training program with Dr. Grof and his associates.

One of the first psychotherapists to pay close attention to breathing patterns in patients was Wilhelm Reich, M. D., an Austrian physician, who at the age of twenty-three had been a disciple of Sigmund Freud in Vienna. Although Freud initially considered Reich one of the most brilliant and capable of the psychoanalysts associated with him, this changed rapidly when Reich began to develop his own ideas, theories, and practices. These became far more related to bodily and biological processes than was consistent with Freud's views. In many respects Reich was one of the first holistic psychotherapists in his conviction that the mind and body were identical in function though different in form. Reich emigrated to the United States in 1939 and became the leader of a school of therapy. Alexander Lowen, M. D., formerly a student of Wilhelm Reich, developed Bioenergetic Analysis. This is a body-oriented psychotherapy that works vigorously with the body, including breathing, to resolve emotional problems.

In most of the books that have been written on rebirthing a significant portion has also been devoted to the value of "Affirmations" and methods for working with them. Although not all rebirthers necessarily work with affirmations, the combination of rebirthing and affirmations is an effective blend. Sondra Ray and Leonard Orr are among proponents for the use and practice of affirmations. Affirmations are declarations expressed in the present tense to achieve desired goals. While they are not a new "invention," modern versions and new techniques have evolved in recent decades.

14

Affirmations

There is an often quoted saying, "War is too important to leave to the generals." This is also true about health and some aspects of illness. There is an increasingly large place for methods individuals can carry out by themselves, given some instruction and guidance. This need not diminish the role of physicians, surgeons, and psychotherapists. This applies to nutrition, exercise, personal growth, and spiritual development.

I am impressed with how much is possible, and is available, for anyone to help themselves in a variety of ways for healing and for growth. I have spent a large part of my professional career as a psychotherapist. I have also spent time and money as a "client" or patient in psychotherapy at different times in my life. Psychotherapy usually emphasizes the need for a trained person or expert to help the other one who cannot find solutions without significant assistance. This remains true, but it can obscure how much a person might accomplish on their own.

The use of affirmations is one such technique that can sometimes achieve dramatic results. I discovered the power of affirmations only in recent years. It was initially easy for me to dismiss such a process, since it is based on mental or intellectual processes, in contrast to dealing with emotional states. It had taken me several decades to overcome my attachment to the intellect and to discover the importance and power of the emotions, especially when they are unconscious, as I had learned in theory from my earlier Freudian training. This was reinforced in later studies and therapy, which dealt more directly with emotional release techniques. Overcoming intellectual rigidities and a previous overemphasis on mental processes could sometimes lead me or others to play down intellectual activity, including the use of reason and thinking.

As I learned about affirmations and how to use them, I found it was tempting at first to be arrogant toward the apparent simplicity of the process, and without a theoretical base. Simultaneously, affirmations were contrary to logical, rational thinking. This suggests that sometimes there can be nothing as irrational as rational thinking. As with many activities already described in previous chapters, there may not be "scientific proof" and yet many people can readily report, "it works."

Affirmations do work. Initially the experience and the results can look magical, or silly, and clearly not logical. Some assumptions for why they work may be related more to metaphysical or spiritual principles than to ordinary laws of physics or conventional psychology. If so, so be it. Other explanations may not relate to conventional and familiar schools of psychology. Nonetheless there is the reality of results.

A clinician or physician may be more skeptical about the use and effectiveness of affirmations, since the emphasis of their training and practice is on what is wrong, disturbing, pathological, in need of correction or cure. The clinical viewpoint has a built-in pessimism, since it is necessarily concerned with what is wrong or problematic. Philosophically this often conveys a sense of helplessness, being at the mercy of uncontrollable forces, both internal and external.

I am not proposing a denial of unconscious factors outside ordinary awareness, nor the force of external elements. Still, there are other viewpoints that are less pessimistic, declaring that conscious elements of the mind and personality can be drawn on in the service of emotional and physical healing, also for personal growth and spiritual enlightenment. The history of Sigmund Freud's psychoanalysis, almost a century old, includes the history of colleagues who became dissenters and developed their separate theories and practices. One of them was Otto Rank. I mentioned him earlier as the author of a book on Birth Trauma. He developed a theory that anxiety is rooted in the traumas of birth. He called his system Will Therapy. (His writings are acknowledged, even by those devoted to his teachings, to be almost impossible to read.) He did have an influence on some later leaders of the Human Potential Movement in the United States in the 1960s and 1970s. He believed that a person was not a victim of his unconscious instinctual forces but could direct these forces, and had the potential for shaping them for creative self-expression and growth. Another positive aspect to his views was his influence on two American graduate schools of social work, after he came to the United States in the 1930s. His influence was a stimulus for time-limited therapy and counseling. Rank believed in the ability of individuals to make choices despite their handicaps or immaturity, as with young children. One of his students, later a professor of social work at the University of Pennsylvania School of Social Work, wrote a book, *The Nature of Choice in Casework Process*, derived from Rank's ideas.

Another innovative dissenter in the early years of psychoanalysis was Roberto Assagioli, M.D. of Venice, Italy. In 1910 he began to elaborate theories and techniques for expanding personality, contributing to personal growth and leading to higher states of consciousness. Although he was the first to introduce psychoanalysis into Italy, he decided that he preferred integration to analysis, and thus called his work, *Psychosynthesis*. By 1927 he had broken away from psychoanalysis entirely. He did not write about his views until 1965. He sought to develop a science of the self, and its energies. He also used the concept of Will, not as the commonly used "willpower" but as part of the Self, or Higher Self, in a more spiritual sense.

One of Dr. Assagioli's former students, Martha Crampton, Director of the Canadian Institute of Psychosynthesis, wrote about psychological energy transformations (Crampton, 1974) by commenting, "Energy follows thought." She was describing how to convert imperfections and weaknesses into the opposite qualities and attitudes. She mentioned one method in Psychosynthesis is a technique based on the principle of substitution. She wrote:

> These approaches do not attempt to convert negative into positive energy directly, but do so indirectly by replacing the negative thought, attitude, or assumption with the opposite positive thought. Their effectiveness is based on the fact that the negative attitude tends to be "starved out" through lack of attention and that the effect of the opposite positive attitude which is actively cultivated is to counteract or cancel out the corresponding negative attitude.

Crampton then refers to one type of substitution technique as "affirmation—replacing the negative thought with a corresponding positive thought. It is a simple technique for a person to use, though some skill is required in formulating an effective affirmation." Assagioli described the use of affirmations in what he called "The technique of evocative words" (Assagioli, 1965).

The Power of Positive Thinking by Rev. Norman Vincent Peale was a best-seller for several decades in the United States and Canada, easily ignored by clinicians but avidly read by the public. He did not elaborate detailed techniques for affirmations but he obviously encouraged people to find ways to overcome some of their fears and personal problems. There is more to affirmations than simply being or thinking positively.

Leonard Orr, the developer of Rebirthing, or Conscious Connected Breathing, has also developed specific ways for working with affirmations. Sondra Ray has elaborated these techniques in detail in her several books.

For the past four years my wife and I have given two-hour workshops on the use of affirmations. In these we have taught the participants how to use affirmations in their daily lives.

As Jean recently commented to me as I was preparing this chapter, "It is a tangible, mechanical tool, nothing airy-fairy at all." Louise L. Hay, who refers to herself as a metaphysical counselor, has written several excellent self-help books that include extensive use of affirmations. In her highly readable book, *You Can Heal Your Life* (Hay, 1984), she comments, "Consistently used affirmations become beliefs and will always produce results, sometimes in ways we cannot even imagine." I have heard it said, "Be careful what you ask for! You may get it."

I shall present the gist of what we usually teach in our two-hour workshop, so that you can learn enough to start creating your own affirmations. The definition of an affirmation is "a positive thought that you choose to immerse in your consciousness to produce a desired result." (Orr & Ray, 1977). Another definition is "Affirmations are controlled thoughts." A third definition that we have used is: "Affirmations are creating an attitude to make a change in physical reality." Before describing specifically how to design an appropriate positive affirmation, it is necessary first to decide what it is a person wishes to achieve. This may be either the elimination of a negative thought, attitude, or experience, or to obtain something they believe they don't have, or an increase in what they have. There are no limitations to goals.

To make the idea and the process simple, we often suggest that affirmations are useful for finding a parking place in a busy area of a town or city. If this hadn't worked for me many dozens of times since I first tried it, I might hesitate to describe it. The truth is that it has worked for me at least ninety-five percent of the time. I am in no way suggesting that it is magical or that it defies any ordinary laws of nature. It is recommended that a person write an affirmation on a three by five card, stating "I, ———, always find a parking-place for my car." This can be used at any time of the day, including noontime in front of the post-office. Saying it and thinking it are also helpful. As you approach where you wish to park, you begin to look for your place. The person who is not expecting to find a place manages not to see an open spot, since they are noticing other things. One operating principle is that the mind doesn't like to be wrong. If you are sure you won't or can't expect to find a spot, you can be sure you won't. The positive expectation will therefore result in a greater likelihood that: the space is there. Sometimes it is necessary to make another trip around the block before "your place" is there for you. The irrational truth is that you will usually find a place. The pure rationalist will insist it is merely coincidence. The Jungian will say it is an example of synchronicity, or a non-connecting principle. An agnostic can comfortably say, "I don't understand but I am glad it is there for me." Some of us will merely say, "Of course. Why not?" Anyhow, using this kind of affirmation is handy. At times a part of me remains somewhat skeptical, but I find no danger in using the technique.

On one occasion I drove into the middle of New York City, in Manhattan, to visit the only store in Manhattan that sells recorders (wooden flutes) and recorder music. I affirmed to myself and to my driving companions that I would find a place to park close to the store. I drove off the West Side Drive onto a large cross-street at Seventy-second Street and found a spot about five car lengths before Broadway. The store was less than half a block around the corner! This is not proof of anything at all, but it was highly gratifying.

More important affirmations can be created for any kind of personal psychological, physical, or spiritual difficulty. It has frequently been used for personal relationship problems, such as for someone who struggles to maintain or find a close love relationship, or for someone who has low self-esteem. Many people have a strong inner conviction, "I'm not good enough," or "I never get my share." Thoughts become beliefs, which then become perceptions. This leads to the experiences that continually reinforce these perceptions.

It may often feel uncanny how true it is that the experience of the believer reflects the inner conviction or belief. Such a person might write a positive affirmation, "I am going to have a satisfying job." It is important to write the affirmation always in the present tense, even though it is to obtain some desired goal not yet experienced but sought for. "I am going to. . ." keeps the goal always in the future. To create the future, it is necessary, therefore, to use the present tense, declaring, "I have a satisfying job."

To avoid any negative tone an affirmation should not have words like "I no longer smoke." For reasons that are unclear, the unconscious mind hears the negative word "no" louder than the rest of the statement, and it may have no effect on the behavior. Using a positive present-tense affirmation, "I have clear, healthy lungs" increases the probability of being free of the smoking habit. Using this affirmation may require several months of steady work for results. With many affirmations the truth is often that the person already has what they are seeking to have or be in the future. This can be particularly true concerning personal attributes.

If a person in a workshop at first cannot find something that they wish to have, do, or be in a positive way, we suggest they might start with a general affirmation, such as "I am grateful for————," or "It is O.K. for————to————." They can fill the blanks with whatever occurs to them. After a person has written an affirmation in a positive way in the present tense, such as "I have an abundance of money," they are asked to write it on a sheet of paper, with a vertical line near the right side of the paper, with the heading of "Response" at the top. Then they write the affirmation on a line or two to the left. After writing the affirmation, they then write a word or two as a comment. At first they may find it so contrary to their present situation that it is easy to write "nonsense" on one line. Then they write it again on the next line, and to the right again write a response, which might be "no way" or "crazy." They continue to write the same affirmation and a response after it as often as is necessary for it to sound less peculiar. Often the charge or reaction decreases, and the person may find they are willing or can write "perhaps" or "why not?"

The next step is to write the affirmation on a piece of paper or a card in the first person, such as "I, John, am an outgoing person." It is essential to include one's first name. This makes the affirmation highly specific, and reinforces the connection between the individual and their affirmation. Like a written signature, it is theirs and theirs alone. "I, John, am an outgoing person" might be an affirmation written by someone who feels shy with people and would like to be more outgoing and relaxed with people. This is then repeated two more times in the first person, and then it is written in the second person, as "You, John, are an outgoing person." Many of the negative views that a person has come from childhood when they were told that they were a certain way that sounded critical. This also is written for a total of three times, and then in the third person, as if others were talking about him; "He, John, is an outgoing person." Then for the tenth line a final first person statement is written, "I, John, am an outgoing person."

These ten lines comprise a SET. One can benefit writing them every day and writing as many sets as there is time available. We inform the workshop participants that the repetitive use of the affirmation will simultaneously make its impression on the person's mind and erase the old thought pattern, producing permanent desirable changes in their life. Old cliches can be entirely correct: "Nothing succeeds like success."

Unfortunately the opposite can freqently be true or become a truth for some people, so they become convinced that they are doomed to failure because they have experienced failure. Thinking and belief can be changed. A key ingredient that we emphasize is Intention. No one can make another person change. They can only encourage or offer ways to do so. Choice is a critical part of the process.

To make the affirmations work for a person, there are several mechanical procedures that increase their effectiveness. The first advice we list for a person is to work with only one or two at a time, and not try to do too many at once. Some people find that they may create a list of seven or eight. After they have worked on one or two to their satisfaction, they can proceed down the list. Occasionally, they discover that some of the others have already occurred without directly working on them.

The next advice is to write each affirmation ten to twenty times, including the first, second, and third person statements as mentioned already. It also helps to say them aloud for five minutes three times a day. Making a tape recording and playing it back also can reinforce the process. Looking in a mirror as you say them to yourself also can aid the process. Saying them to a friend is another method that can be added or used instead of saying them to yourself. Have a friend say your affirmation back to you. It becomes even more powerful when your ears hear another voice saying your affirmation to you. Writing them on notes that are left around, on the mirror in the bathroom, bedroom, or on a car dashboard, helps. All this is continued until they are totally integrated.

We further suggest that an affirmation to find a parking place is a good one to start with, since it usually increases further motivation to work on others more complex or apparently more difficult. Begin gently and not too grandiosely. It is best to use whatever is one's mother tongue. If one has moved from a native country to another and now speaks in a different language, it can be helpful to write and speak the affirmation in the original mother tongue. If a person has had a childhood nickname, it sometimes works better to use that name than one's adult name. This is better because the old messages and attitudes that you are trying to overcome are harvested from seeds sown in childhood.

One exercise we use in our workshop is to give each person a sheet of positive affirmations, and ask them to read the list. If there is any one or several that ring a bell, or jangle the mind or cause the person to flinch, they are advised to put a checkmark next to it, and consider using that as one to practice. The list we use is as follows:

* I am lovable.
* It's safe to be loved.
* I love being alive.
* The more I enjoy life, the better life gets.
* I think highly of myself in the presence of others.
* I am good enough.
* I am successful.
* I am intelligent.
* I always give myself what I need.
* All my relationships are successful.
* People want me to win.
* I am self-confident.
* I express myself well.
* I have abundance.
* I make money easily.
* My body mirrors my inner beauty.
* My body vibrates with health and vitality.
* I am strong and joyfully alive.
* The more beauty I see in others, the more beautiful I become.

The term, affirmation, usually suggests a positive thought. There are, of course, negative affirmations, which may be beliefs or comments that a person is not aware of, because they have lived with them for so long that they are second nature to the person. A person says, "I'm so clumsy!" without even hearing themselves say it. If asked if they heard what they just said, they may not be able to repeat it until their attention is forcibly called to it. Even when they recognize it, they speak of it as if it were an inevitable truth. It had become so for them. Instead of "Seeing is believing," they have reversed the equation to "believing is seeing," as Wayne Dyer has titled his book. It might be useful for a "clumsy" person to work on an affirmation that states: "I am always graceful and well-coordinated." The challenge for many people is to tolerate giving up old patterns or beliefs, even if they are self-destructive or hurtful. Change can be scary for some, or at least anxiety-provoking. Self-approval and self-acceptance is central to feeling better and happier. Louise Hay comments, "The more you dwell on what you don't want, the more of it you create. The things about yourself or your life that you have always disliked are probably still with you." The corollary to this is that you get what you concentrate on.

In the workshop we also briefly quote from the traditional Kahuna philosophy of ancient Hawaii, which also resembles many other metaphysical and spiritual teachings. Four principles from the Kahunas are:

1. You create your own reality.
2. You get what you concentrate on.
3. You are unlimited.
4. Your moment of power is now.

The rest of the workshop is spent practicing on the creation of personal affirmations, and answering questions as enrollees work on the exact phrasing. We also give a brief list of books that contain details on working with affirmations. These are by Sondra Ray and Louise Hay.

On one occasion we were asked to give the workshop as a fifty-minute presentation at a one day conference on holistic health in a nearby university. We did not think that this would be the most satisfactory way to do it, but we decided (and affirmed) that it was possible. When we finished, we could not tell if the audience of twenty people had grasped what we had presented in a short time.

A few months later a couple came to one of our other workshops that we presented closer to home. The husband was an engineer who had been troubled for many years since childhood with nail-biting. He could not stop it, despite several attempts. They reported that they had been at our university lecture, and that the husband had applied the techniques of affirmation. He proudly showed us his fingernails that were normal and attractive, without any signs of having been bitten. He reported that he had been able to stop the habit and had experienced no difficulty for the past several months.

There are always exceptions to rules. I stated that the person has to write or develop their own affirmation. It is possible that someone else can write one and give it to another person. There still remains the choice to use it or discard it, as one sees fit. I was given one several years ago that I continue to use and appreciate. It was given to me under somewhat unusual circumstances. My wife and I attended the annual Maine Healing Arts Festival for the first time. One activity available was a firewalk across a bed of hot coals.

I had not intended to participate in the fire walk initially. I had accompanied my wife to it, to give her moral support, since she had previously witnessed similar fire walks elsewhere, and was considering doing this one. Part of preparation for it included a discussion by the couple who were in charge of it. They also asked anyone who was not going to participate in the actual fire walk, but had attended the discussion, to take off their shoes and socks, roll up their pants, and walk outside in the dark around the bed of coals that had been raked out into a path. This was to be a form of support to those who were participating in the fire walk. As I walked outside and saw five or six of the group walk across the bed of coals, I decided at that moment to do likewise. The others all seemed to me to be ordinary people, in the best sense of the word, and I decided and hoped that I was also. No one in the group of about forty people who walked experienced any burns or blisters. No one appeared to be in any kind of altered state or trance. Many participants, including my wife and myself, walked across the bed of coals a second time, as if we needed to confirm in our mind that we had indeed done it.

The experience was not only an unusual one, but "mind-boggling." There had been nothing in my upbringing or American cultural environment that prepared me for this type of event. There are several detailed accounts written by Americans who have described this in detail, and I shall not attempt to elaborate on it. My point for outlining my experience relates to what happened after the fire walk.

The participants all gathered indoors afterward. The leaders handed out three by five inch file cards, and asked us each to write, as a form of affirmation: "Tonight, September 6, 1987, I walked on fire. I can do anything I choose to do." They then asked each of us to sign our card, and keep it. I have it tacked up on my personal bulletin board. I have further reinforced the statement by fire walking again in two successive years. Perhaps fire walking is a form of affirmation in action. It is not as remarkable a feat as it sounds, except the choosing to do it, overcoming the initial fear, and taking the first step. The rest is easy. The written card with the affirmation is as important to me as the act itself. Together they suggest that we are all much more capable of achieving goals than we sometimes believe.

Practicing the use of affirmations can sensitize a person to hearing themselves or others using negative statements that can operate exactly like hypnotic suggestions. What you say to yourself in the moment that you wake up in the morning may create how your day goes. Often a person scarcely realizes that they have just said silently or aloud, "It's going to be a rough day." How often you have heard someone say, "I got out of the wrong side of the bed." The whole day that follows may be less than a pleasant one, a self-fulfilling, if not satisfying prophecy. Being near a pessimist frequently risks acquiring uncheerful thoughts or feelings.

Affirmations are not the cure or answer for all the ills and problems that people experience. Nonetheless, the power of affirmations can be startling when adequately practiced.

15

Visualization, Guided Imagery and Meditation

Visualization is seeing "with the mind's eye." The use of one's imagination is a process of creating visual images within, imaging. In speaking of affirmations, I quoted Martha Crampton as saying, "energy follows thought." This is equally true with the use of imagery. There is sufficient scientific evidence to demonstrate that the process of imaging occurs mostly in the right side of the brain, and does not require or involve speech. There is also extensive scientific research that shows a clear connection between the creating of images and changes in bodily processes. There can be effects on white cells and other cellular and organ systems.

A forerunner of imagery application is a process developed by a German psychiatrist and neurologist, Dr. Johannes Schultz, in 1930 and further elaborated by Wolfgang Luthe. Dr. Schultz developed a relaxation process he called *Autogenic Training,* a system of mental exercises that included visualizing different parts of the body becoming increasingly relaxed. It was applied in the treatment of stress-related disorders. The process had some similarities to hypnosis and meditation. To practice it required training the patient. Autogenic training also contributed to the development of biofeedback techniques in the 1960s.

Jeanne Achterberg has decribed in detail the role of imagery in healing (Achterberg, 1985) and its roots in shamanism in native cultures throughout the world over the centuries. Shamans are a special type of witch doctor or medicine man, who use imagination in healing extensively. The shamanic tradition is at least twenty thousand years old. Its goals were not necessarily to prevent death, and often dealt with spiritual concerns, to protect the soul. Achterberg has also documented the scientific studies that show the value of visualization and guided imagery. Visualization has become in the past two decades a more vigorously applied practice than previously. Roberto Assagioli, M.D. in 1930 used imagery in Psychosynthesis, and present-day Psychosynthesis therapists make active use of imagery. Carl Jung called it *Active Imagination*. A French psychologist, Robert Desoille, in the 1930s developed what he called "Directed Waking Dream" that involved extensive use of imagery. He continued his explorations into the 1960s.

A contemporary of Robert Desoille, Mme. Colette Aboulker-Muscat, has practiced his method of visual imagery in Jerusalem, Israel since 1954 to the present. In 1974 a New York psychoanalyst and psychiatrist, Gerald Epstein, M. D. met her and was profoundly moved by the results she could achieve with patients. He then spent the next nine years learning from her. After fifteen years of using visualizations in his clinical practice, Dr. Epstein wrote the details of the visualizations he had learned or developed for both emotional and physical problems in *Healing Visualizations: Creating Health Through Imagery* (Epstein, 1989). It is a clear and practical manual for visualization work. The visualizations are brief, easy to follow and apply to over seventy-five physical and emotional disturbances. Dr. Epstein has also written a more technical and detailed book for psycho-spiritual exploration, *Waking Dream Therapy*.

The use of imagery cannot easily be credited to any specific individuals, since it has been applied in many different circumstances, by metaphysical writers, physicians, psychologists, and laypersons. The use of visualization for healing of physical illness or improving physical health is a newer and still controversial development in conventional medicine. Michael Samuels, M. D. presented the use of visualization for physical healing in *The Well Body Book* (Samuels, 1973) and *Seeing with the Mind's Eye* (Samuels & Samuels, 1975). Irving Oyle, D. O. has also described the active use of imagery in physical healing in *The Healing Mind* and *Time Space and the Mind* (Oyle, 1975, 1976).

The most provocative and challenging program using imagery has been the work of Carl Simonton, M. D., a radiation oncologist who has developed a program called *The Simonton Method*. I first read of his ideas in 1972. He had presented his findings and methods at the Academy of Medicine and Parapsychology in Los Angeles, California. The title of his paper was, "The Role of Mind in Cancer Therapy." He described what he had recently started to offer some of his severely ill cancer patients besides radiation therapy. He began to have them do visualization of their cancer and the treatment, along with some techniques for relaxation. He found that some patients lived longer than expected, and had a better quality of life. A few actually experienced remission of their previously diagnosed terminal cancer.

Dr. Simonton and his former wife, Stephanie Matthews-Simonton, developed a program for helping cancer patients improve their chances for recovery with the use of visualization and psychotherapy, both individual and group. They reported about this program in *Getting Well Again* (Simonton, Simonton & Creighton, 1978) and *The Healing Family* (Matthews-Simonton, 1984) The Simontons have each developed a center for conducting their programs in California and Texas. Conventional medicine has not accepted the validity of their work, since there have not been acceptable research documents that are statistically valid. Nonetheless, many patients throughout the United States and England have used Dr. Simonton's methods. Fritjof Capra describes Dr. Simonton's work and ideas in a vivid and informal manner in *Uncommon Wisdom: Conversations with Remarkable People* (Capra, 1988).

Another physician who has included guided imagery in his program for the enhancement of the treatment of cancer is Bernard Siegel, M. D., the author of *Love, Medicine and Miracles* (Siegel, 1986) and *Peace, Love. and Healing* (Siegel, 1989). Dr. Siegel created an organization called ECaP (Exceptional Cancer Patients) in 1978 after he heard the Simontons present their program at a workshop. I visited Dr. Siegel's office in New Haven in 1980 and observed first-hand the group meetings he had started. I shall discuss this in the next chapter on support groups. Dr. Siegel encouraged his patients to use visualization as an adjunct to whatever cancer treatment they were undergoing, or for use post-operatively. He also led patients in guided imagery. This consisted of a person listening to the directions for creating images in their mind and following the "trip" as verbalized. In the back of Dr. Siegel's two books there are guided visualizations that he refers to as "meditations." Dr. Siegel has also recorded audio cassettes of these guided visualizations, and are available through the ECaP organization. Many other tapes are available for meditation and guided imagery by other physicians, psychologists and metaphysical writers.

At a support group meeting for people with serious illnesses at which my wife and I were present, a young woman reported that she had attended a workshop on Creative Visualization several days earlier. Her husband had been diagnosed with AIDS and she herself is HIV-positive. For nearly six months she had been bothered by a hard, painful lymph node in her groin. The lump was the size of a walnut. Her doctors had advised no treatment. She was told it was part of the "progression of the disease."

During the visualization workshop, the leader had the group imagine they were walking across a meadow into a forest. (This was the young woman's first experience at following a directed visualization.) As she described her imagined walk, she said she found the forest "very dark and scary." She had trouble entering it but "a little girl," whom she recognized as herself when she was young, took her by the hand and told her she was safe. She went further into the forest until she came upon an opening in the trees.

In the little glen was a bright ray of light shining down from the sky. She reported that she felt strongly drawn toward the light but felt terrified of it. The little girl holding her hand kept tugging at her and saying to her," It's O.K. Walk into the beam. You'll be safe." With much coaxing, she walked into the beam of golden light.

The young woman reported further that she stepped into the beam of light (in her imagination and visualization). At that point she said she experienced and felt as if she "came apart into little pieces and then came back together again." She then went home after this visualization workshop feeling tired. She fixed supper for her family, and then went to bed early.

When she woke up the next morning she was astonished to find that the lump that had been present for so many months was no longer there. Coincidence? Perhaps, but her participation in the healing visualization during the workshop the day before might have had some influence on her new level of health. Nearly a year later she is still asymptomatic.

Garrett Porter has presented an even more dramatic report of the use of visualization (Porter & Norris, 1985). In September of 1978, when he was nine years old, he was diagnosed with an inoperable brain tumor, an astrocytoma. After a course of as much radiation as was considered medically safe, his clinical symptoms continued to progress. His left leg was affected and other parts of the left side of his body. He was given some biofeedback training by Dr. Steven Fahrion of the Menninger Clinic in Topeka, Kansas. At the same time his parents gave him a tape made by the Simontons. Garrett's grandmother had died of cancer earlier in the year and his parents had obtained the tape for her during her illness. After awhile Garrett found the tape "too boring for a kid." He was then introduced to Dr. Patricia Norris at the Menninger Clinic, to see if she might work with him using visualization and imagery. As Dr. Norris describes in *Why Me?*, she had worked as a clinical psychologist before coming to Topeka, where her parents, Elmer and Alyce Green, had established a well-known research center on biofeedback and voluntary controls of involuntary functions. Dr. Norris also studied Psychosynthesis and was familiar with Carl Simonton's work. She had used imagery techniques with prisoners, and had an interest to work with someone with cancer.

Garrett created his own cassettes for guided imagery and worked on developing his own set of images. In February of 1979 his tumor was seen on CT scan to have grown considerably but no further radiation treatment could be given. It was thought that he had less than one year to live. The details of his fight for his life are vividly described in *Why Me?: Harnessing the Healing Power of the Human Spirit* by Patricia Norris and Garrett Porter (Porter & Norris, 1985).

In February of 1980 he underwent a CT scan because of some symptoms that concerned his pediatrician. A few months earlier Garrett had reported that he did not see the tumor in his own visualizations of his brain. The CT scan showed no signs of any tumor, except a pea-sized fragment of calcification. As reported in *Why Me?*, "The doctor said if he hadn't known better, he would have thought it was surgically removed." As far as I am aware there was no recurrence over the following ten years.

A reading of *Why Me?* does not suggest that it was visualization work alone that contributed to Garrett Porter's healing. He had several highly supportive people as a network that sustained and encouraged him throughout his ordeals and triumphs. Not only strong family support but also others, including a telephone network of new friends. The term, support, means far more than merely keeping up a person's spirits in a time of stress.

Meditation: Until the 1960s, few Americans were familiar with spiritual traditions such as Buddhism, Zen Buddhism, and some aspects of Yoga or other Hindu traditions of India. It is less well-known that meditation has played a part in the Christian and Jewish mystical traditions. Mysticism itself has gathered a mixed reputation over the centuries in the prevailing religious traditions of the West and Near East. This has happened because the mystic often experiences religious inspiration without benefit of clergy, which leads to suspicions of heresy. For various reasons, therefore, many citizens initially feel frightened or at least cautious about meditation, until they learn more about it, and can appreciate that it is not contrary to any set of religious teachings. Many non-religious persons also can learn meditation purely for stress reduction and relaxation, without needing to incorporate it into a spiritual path.

The best known form of meditation in the United States has been *Transcendental Meditation*, or TM, introduced in the early 1960s by Maharishi Mahesh Yogi and his students. It has also been the subject of more than twenty years of research by scientists more extensively than any other form of meditation. Herbert Benson, M. D. has written several books on "The Relaxation Response" (Benson, 1975) in which he describes a method for obtaining improved mental and physical functioning, derived from meditative practices, free of any spiritual connotations. In a later book, *Beyond the Relaxation Response* (Benson, 1984), Dr. Benson speaks of the "Faith Factor," or a combination of an individual's deepest personal beliefs combined with the relaxation response. He presents evidence and explanation for why this combination can "help an individual reach enhanced states of health and well-being."

Lawrence LeShan, Ph. D. is a psychologist who has contributed in several ways to better understanding and methods for improving health and healing. He has written an excellent guide to meditation in *How to Meditate* (LeShan, 1974). He describes a wide range of meditative styles, derived from several spiritual and religious traditions. The practice of meditation also can help in using visualization and guided imagery more effectively, since meditation is a process that allows a person to develop skills and experience in "going inward."

Physiological studies have shown the positive effects of meditation on lowering blood pressure, decreasing anxiety, and having other longterm effects on both psychological and physiological processes. Although I had learned some simple forms of meditation in 1972 from a colleague who used it in her group therapy with patients, I had never followed it as a consistent and regular discipline until 1990. Then I began to practice meditation on a regular basis. I have usually practiced it for twenty minutes twice a day.

After about two months I happened to check my blood pressure, which had never been elevated, and had usually measured about 120/80 to 125/85. Any reading under 140/90 is normal. The reading at this time was 115/65. I was startled and repeated it, and it remained the same. At first I thought the machine might be defective, and I couldn't understand why it was lower. Then I realized I had been doing regular meditation for two months and this might well be the explanation. This lowered reading has continued over the following year and a half.

There are some individuals who do experience more anxiety when meditating rather than less. This is unusual but not improbable. To let go of the mind's thoughts and "empty the mind" can provoke uneasiness in some. Yet, most people experience meditation as a calming, peaceful experience that can do no harm and can offer many benefits. Joan Borysenko, Ph. D. speaks of meditation producing "stress hardiness" as a contribution of meditation (Borysenko, 1987). She defines meditation as "any activity that keeps the attention pleasantly anchored in the present moment." She also describes a simple way to meditate in "Minding the Body, Mending the Mind."

The University of Massachusetts Medical Center operates a Stress Reduction Clinic directed by Jon Kabat-Zinn, Ph. D. Dr. Zinn has helped over four thousand medical patients over the past twelve years in the clinic's eight-week stress reduction program for stress, pain and illness. One major component of this program is the use of a type of meditation called *Mindfulness Meditation*. This form of meditation is many centuries old and is a part of the Buddhist tradition. Its use is an excellent example of East meeting West. The methods are applicable to Westerners who need not follow any religious or spiritual teachings to make use of it. Dr. Kabat-Zinn describes in detail the entire program that he uses at the Stress Reduction Clinic in his *Full Catastrophe Living* (Kabat-Zinn, 1990). The subtitle of the book is "Using the Wisdom of Your Body and Mind to Face Stress, Pain and Illness."

The practice of meditation is particularly useful in the United States and other industrialized countries for those persons who are constantly "on the run" or working under a sense of pressure, dead-lines, or simply driving in commuter traffic every day. (I do not recommend meditation while driving.) Stress plays a significant role in so many diseases of industrialized countries, that techniques for stress reduction are critically important. Meditation is clearly among the most useful.

16

Support Groups

Ever since the ancient Greeks journeyed to the sacred healing shrines at Epidaurus and Cos and joined with others, people have found help by gathering together in groups. In many traditional or tribal cultures, such as the Navaho Indians of the Southwest United States, there are healing ceremonies conducted by a healer or medicine man. The ill person often undergoes the ceremonies in the presence of the family and the local community, who function as a support system. The communal group participates through group singing, and by their presence give support to the patient. In this process there is still a professional healer and a single patient.

Alcoholics Anonymous is a more modern idea of a group that offers support to every member of the group without specified professionals leading the group. Its founder, often called Bill (Wilson), started AA in the 1930s. He had been troubled with alcoholism. He found that getting together with others helped him to remain sober and stay "on the wagon." Over the decades since he started the first AA group, the AA movement has become a national program. It has been life-saving for many citizens, with a high degree of effectiveness. It is not the only approach to helping people with alcoholism, but it has an excellent record of achievement. Following the same pattern, there is also *Narcotics Anonymous* for drug users.

The field of Social Work has contributed to the development of many kinds of groups, usually led or directed by a trained professional. This is also true in the fields of clinical psychology and psychiatry. Group therapy is an accepted form of treatment for many problems with which people are struggling. Its use for help with physical illnesses is less common. With the development of humanistic psychology and the Human Potential Movement in the 1960s and 1970s in the United States, there has been an interest in groups without leaders. When I attended the summer workshops of the American Academy of Psychotherapists throughout the 1960s, a popular activity among members was the "leaderless group." There were also other leader-directed or chaired groups. The leaderless ones consisted of psychotherapists sharing their personal thoughts and feelings. The participants found the meetings meaningful and therapeutic. The goal was not to learn new techniques nor acquire professional knowledge. They were intense and emotional in the honesty of the sharing. I vividly recall one man sharing about an acute crisis in his life that had occurred almost thirty years earlier when he was in college. He had become seriously ill and had to return home, not knowing what was wrong with him. Shortly afterward he was operated on for a brain abscess. In the group session he shared that he had never discussed this highly upsetting experience with his psychoanalyst, when he had been in therapy some years later. As he shared the story, he let go of an agonized sob that apparently had been sitting inside him for many years, but never expressed in his previous psychotherapy. In these leaderless groups there was no hierarchy and no sense of anyone having to be helped or treated.

I am not suggesting that leaderless groups are better, but only that they clearly can make a contribution. There may often be a need for someone to be a gentle referee or "housekeeper" of some basic rules. More organized groups often have a facilitator, or two co-facilitators, to function in this way, without any obligation to be experts. Some health organizations that are public service organizations, such as the American Cancer Society, the American Leukemia Society, and other similar organizations have sponsored support groups. The American Cancer Society has developed *Can Surmount* and *I Can Cope* programs for people living with cancer. For more than a decade the American Leukemia Society has sponsored The Candlelighters, which is an organization for the parents of children with leukemia. There are also grass-roots organizations that have developed for citizens with health problems.

In 1974 Orville Kelley of Burlington, Iowa started one or the first groups organized to help cancer patients. He had been diagnosed in 1973 with lymphocytic lymphosarcoma. (He also was an "Atomic" veteran, present at the atomic bomb testings in the 1950s in Nevada.) Kelley had invited a group of other cancer patients to meet and discuss the impact of cancer on their lives, and to explore what they could do to reestablish a sense of joy in their lives despite their illness. From these meetings a national organization, Make Today Count, developed, and is still active with chapters in cities throughout the United States. The meetings are not limited to persons with cancer, but for anyone who is dealing with a potentially life-threatening disease.

I attended several meetings of a Make Today Count group in Connecticut in 1980. It was my first awareness of the paradox that a group of people facing a possibly shortened life span could be as cheerful and up-beat as they were. Both the positive mood of each person and the group spirit were impressive. Although I was there as a quiet observer without any health problems, I felt cheered up and encouraged by the experience. People experience the news that they have a serious and possibly life-threatening disease with a range of emotions and reactions. For those who do not remain totally overwhelmed, and do not feel helpless and hopeless, there can be a spiritual awakening, or reawakening, which sharpens their appreciation of life itself, and may move them to find purpose and meaning in life, for whatever length may be remaining. This spiritual quality can be felt by others. Elizabeth Kubler-Ross, M. D. has commented on this in detail.

Dr. Kubler-Ross became the first psychiatrist to study the psychological aspects of death and dying. This is not a subject that had ever appealed to any of her professional colleagues prior to her research. She has worked with thousands of people for the past twenty-five years, before and since the publication of her first book, *On Death and Dying* (Kubler-Ross. 1969). Her attitude is expressed in the subtitle, "What the dying have to teach doctors, nurses, clergy and families."

I had the opportunity in 1985 to participate in one of her five-day workshops titled "Life, Death and Transition." She has led workshops throughout the world, sharing her ideas. She has helped tens of thousands to deal with their personal crises, and some relatives and friends who are close to them. She has also trained many thousands of professionals to deal better with death and dying issues, and deal with losses of any kind, for their clients and for themselves.

Elizabeth Kubler-Ross reported that she has observed that children as much as adults move rapidly through stages of spiritual growth when confronted with a life-threatening illness. It is this quality that sometimes can be observed and experienced in a support group that deals with life-threatening situations. Dr. Kubler-Ross was a major influence that contributed to the development of another large network of support groups throughout the United States and several other countries.

In 1975 Gerald J. Jampolsky, M. D., a child psychiatrist, started a support group for children with serious or life-threatening illnesses. He had gone through several personal crises, which he describes vividly in *Out of Darkness into the Light* (Jampolsky, 1989). A friend sent him an early draft of *A Course in Miracles* (1976), which presented methods for spiritual transformation. Because of his working with this material, he found answers to most of his personal issues at the time. A small group of friends and he started a weekly meeting of students of the *Course*. Part of the process was to listen for "inner guidance." He experienced this later in 1975.

A short time before, he had accompanied another physician on the doctor's ward rounds as he visited an eight-year-old boy with serious cancer. The boy asked his doctor, "What's it like to die?" The doctor changed the subject. In thinking about that visit afterward, Dr. Jampolsky reports, "it occurred to me that children like him need a safe haven to be heard and to talk about their concerns. Perhaps here was an area of unmet need where I could be helpful." He further states that the idea came to him like an inner dictation, which included a vision for starting what became the Center for Attitudinal Healing in Tiburon, California.

In March of 1980 I heard Dr. Jampolsky and six of the children from the Center present their experiences, at a conference on healing. By this time there had been almost five years of Center activity. Most of the children were dealing with profoundly serious diseases. They had been meeting in weekly support groups, led by volunteers who became trained to act as facilitators for the groups. The Center gradually set up separate parent groups and sibling groups. I visited the Center in 1982 and in 1989. By 1989 the Center was conducting more than thirty groups a week, which now included groups for adults and children with AIDs. Also groups for children whose parents were dealing with "catastrophic" illnesses met.

As interested professionals and laypersons from all over the United States and

Canada became interested in the processes developed at the Center for Attitudinal Healing, training courses were established. Other centers have opened in other cities. Although there is no direct sponsorship of these centers by the Tiburon center, they do model themselves after it. The Center began a telephone network that connected one person to another with similar problems, in another part of the country, so that they could share with each other.

Dr. Jampolsky is the author of several books. His first, *Love Is Letting Go of Fear*, is an excellent introduction to the basic principles presented in *Course in Miracles*, and deals particularly with issues of forgiveness. Because of the writings and work of Dr. Jampolsky, the subject of attitudinal healing has become more well-known and many support groups have used the ideas and methods of attitudinal healing. Both Alcoholics Anonymous and support groups based on attitudinal healing have strong spiritual roots. These have not required anyone to put aside their personal religious practices nor adopt any specific form of religious practice. Some citizens with a more negative or disinterested attitude toward religious or spiritual concepts may find this troublesome at times, but the opposite also may occur. A properly conducted support group does not attempt to do any proselytizing of any specific religious viewpoint.

An interesting observation by Dr. Jampolsky has been that each member of a group, such as in the children's support group, is a teacher to everyone else. Even a young child can teach older children and adults about the experience of coping with a life-threatening illness.

ECaP, the Exceptional Cancer Patient organization in New Haven, Connecticut, is another model for support groups. I mentioned it in the previous chapter on visualization. Bernard Siegel, M. D. has been a practicing surgeon for more than twenty years. He also was influenced by Elizabeth Kubler-Ross, M. D. and Carl Simonton, M. D.

In 1978 Dr. Siegel invited his patients with cancer to meet with him in his office. The purpose was to discuss ideas and methods for living more joyfully and perhaps even longer. He discovered that only ten to fifteen percent were willing or could participate in something beyond the usual medical and surgical methods already offered. Despite the small number Dr. Siegel continued to develop a program of support groups. At first he had groups facilitated and guided by a nurse, and later a social worker.

Eventually the program grew, and it obtained volunteers who undertook facilitator training. ECaP became an independent organization with its own building, and both professional and non-professional staff. Dr. Siegel's two books, *Love, Medicine and Miracles* and *Peace, Love and Healing* (Siegel, 1986, 1989) present his philosophy, and methods. Although he has some supporters among the medical profession, he has incurred sharp criticisms for emphasizing the emotional aspects of cancer, particularly as a causative factor, and for treatment. Although in public lectures he makes clear there is no intention to arouse guilt nor blame of anyone with an illness, his writings have sometimes been interpreted to mean that.

Both my wife and I have participated in the training program presently offered by ECaP for anyone interested in facilitating support groups. It is clear and explicit in the material presented that emotional factors are important, but they are not the only issue with which patients must deal. The entire topic of emotional factors in cancer and in other physical illnesses is one that stirs emotional reactions in many physicians and medical educators. The continued scientific focus on cellular and molecular processes appears to move medicine at times further away from the awareness of psychological factors. It also should be mentioned that medical students and residents receive very little training in practical methods for dealing with the emotions and psychosocial aspects of physical illness. It is not a conspiracy, but a major omission, yet to be corrected.

The ECaP program has stimulated many citizens to look for support groups in their local communities. An interesting example of a network of support groups is the H. O. P. E. network in Maine. Kenneth Hamilton, M. D., also a surgeon with more than twenty years of experience, became interested in developing a support group derived from ECaP philosophy. Beginning in 1987 in Norway, Maine, Dr. Hamilton gathered a group of citizens who were living with different life-threatening illnesses. Cancer patients were not the only members, since others with serious physical illnesses also attended. H. O. P. E. stands for Healing of Patients Exceptional. Since the first group was convened, other ones have started. There are presently twelve groups in different communities in Maine, led by facilitators who are trained to conduct such groups. The facilitators meet monthly to review and discuss their groups, and to obtain additional training and support. New groups are developed as citizens in different communities request it, and as facilitators can be made available. Most support groups run by various organizations do not charge regular fees for participation, but depend on donations and fund-raising.

Despite the founding of ECaP and H. O. P. E. by two surgeons, most support groups do not operate as part of medical institutions nor are many mental health professionals involved in working with people with major physical problems. There are trends, however, that are encouraging. There is a recently established field of psycho-oncology, concerned with reseach and the development of psychological methods for helping patients with cancer. Before this there were earlier pioneers who explored the psychological aspects of cancer. These highly experienced psychotherapists have treated cancer patients over the past fifty years, and have presented their observations and results in their various writings. Among the first in this century was Wilhelm Reich, M.D. Reich wrote *The Cancer Biopathy* (Reich, 1973), based on articles he wrote in 1942, and eventually published in 1948. Alexander Lowen, M. D. became a student of Reich and later developed *Bioenergetic Analysis* in 1956. Lowen has written about the application of bioenergetic therapy to cancer in several articles. He has described two patients who were able to obtain a remission of an apparently terminal cancer through the application of a body-oriented type of psychotherapy, bioenergetic analysis.

Another psychotherapist, Dr. Lawrence LeShan, has conducted intensive psychotherapy, beginning in the 1950s, with many patients with advanced cancer. He had one group of patients with advanced cancer achieve an almost fifty percent remission rate. He describes his experiences and his approach in *Cancer as a Turning Point* (LeShan, 1989). This does not mean that patients necessarily seek or often want psychological help. Dr. Bernard Siegel's observations are that only about ten to fifteen percent of patients are willing or able to take a more active responsibility for their treatment. He also estimates that about seventy percent expect and prefer the doctor to do the planning or the treatment without the patient's active participation. In speaking of cancer, Dr. Siegel also reported that about ten or fifteen percent really does not want to survive. This may be related to intrinsic depressive attitudes, or because of the conditions of their physical status.

A newsworthy scientific article appeared in the British medical journal, *The Lancet*, on October 14, 1989. Its senior author, David Spiegel, M. D. is professor of Psychiatry and Behavioral Sciences at Stanford University School of Medicine in California. The title of his paper is "Effect of Psychosocial Treatment on Survival of Patients with Metastatic Breast Cancer" (Spiegel, et al., 1989). It reports on a carefully performed study of the effects of supportive group therapy on the survival rate of a group of patients. Dr. Spiegel elaborated on his findings in a 1991 article in *Advances, The Journal of Mind-Body Health* (Spiegel, 1991) in which he states, "It is worth noting that we did not find that any psychological variables were associated with survival time. It was only participation in the support groups that seemed to make a difference."

As a person committed to the use of scientific methodology, Dr. Spiegel is understandably cautious in his conclusions, although his findings are dramatic. He suggests, "medical research should examine evidence regarding the possibility that mental events affect the course of disease." He presents clear evidence that it is more than a possibility. Many thousands of participants in support groups would agree, and those patients Dr. LeShan and Dr. Lowen had treated successfully. Dr. Spiegel's research with a ten-year follow-up documents this.

The study involved eighty-six women with severe metastatic cancer of the breast. Thirty-six were in a control group who received all the appropriate medical and surgical treatment available at the time. A matching group of fifty women with essentially the same degree of severity of disease, who had received the same types of treatment, attended weekly supportive group therapy and were taught self-hypnosis for pain. After ten years there were only three survivors among the eighty-six women. The three survivors were all in the group of patients assigned to undergo the supportive group therapy. Since these women were all dealing with severe states of cancer, the lengths of survival were measured in months. The control group had an average of eighteen months of survival. Those in the therapy group lived an average of thirty-six months. The patients all had volunteered for the research, and were assigned randomly to either the control group or the experimental group. They were not given any reason to believe that intervention or participation in the supportive group therapy would affect the course of their disease or improve survival time. The goal was to see if the quality of life could be improved.

Dr. Spiegel honestly acknowledges that the original purpose of the study was not to see if survival time could be extended at all, but to see what effects occur on the mood and the pain of women with advanced breast cancer. Although the average survival of the women in the therapy group was thirty-six months, it is important to know that, for those women who attended more than ten sessions, the average survival time increased to forty-one months compared to eighteen months in the control group. Because the findings were surprising, a careful review and extensive rechecking took place.

In reviewing what took place in the therapy group process. Dr. Spiegel states, "When people honestly face their own mortality and make rational choices about how to live their lives, it can have an invigorating effect." Other published studies have clearly shown that social integration—feeling a part of a family or social network— increases life-span. Interestingly a frequent comment made in the H. O. P. E. and ECaP groups is that the group is like a "second family," in the good sense of the word. It is a common experience for many cancer patients that they and their family members are often not able to discuss frankly the facts of the disease, and their feelings, with each other. Family members often feel unsure of what to say or do, for fear of upsetting the patient or themselves. It is often easier for a patient to discuss it in a group with others who are dealing with the same problems and are not relatives. It can be helpful for family members or significant others to attend a support group with the patient, or attend a separate group.

Dr. Spiegel summarizes what these findings mean for patients. He presents five points:

> 1. Support groups can clearly improve the quality of life. We were able to show reduced mood disturbance. They had reduced pain.
>
> 2. It may be that by teaching patients to manage stress better, the patients can learn techniques that allow their bodies valuable resources in fighting illness.
>
> 3. This effect comes not by denying the illness or wishing it away but by more successfully managing one's life in terms of family relationships, relationships with physicians, and one's own feelings about having a serious illness, and dealing with these factors as directly as possible.
>
> 4. There is no evidence that such techniques are a cure for cancer, but there is some evidence that the techniques might prolong life with cancer.
>
> 5. Should future research confirm these findings, it would support a strong recommendation that group support of this type be added to the combined modality treatment as a STAN-DARD [my emphasis] care for patients with metastatic breast cancer."

I asked Dr. Spiegel by telephone why he expressed cautiousness in his last proposal, since his research appeared to me clear in its results. He replied that it is usual in scientific reports, such as in cancer chemotherapy research, to look for repeated studies to confirm the first one. I understand his cautiousness. Nonetheless, I am convinced that inclusion of psychological support for anyone with a serious illness, not only metastatic breast cancer, would be useful This can apply even if the illness is not immediately life-threatening. It would be even more critically needed in the face of life-threatening diseases. It is common for the medical profession generally to refer to some diseases as "terminal." In Dr. Spiegel's group of eighty-six women, three were living ten years later. Statistics declare a certain medical diagnosis as "terminal," as shown in this group of women, and yet it was not possible to decide in advance exactly who would die soon and who might live longer, especially for those who were assigned to the support group.

I have not participated in any organized scientific studies regarding the value of support groups. My observations of several dozens of participants are anecdotal. I have known individuals who have attended a support group for several years, as well as others for shorter periods of time. My observations totally agree with Dr. Spiegel's findings. The cases reported in writings and lectures by Dr. Bernard Siegel and Dr. Carl Simonton also bear witness to this.

Both Dr. Siegel and Dr. Simonton have been criticized severely by medical colleagues for conveying "false hope." Dr. Spiegel refers in *Advances* (Spiegel, 1991), to "wild claims about the powers of the mind." He does acknowledge that it has been media hype that suggests, "people can wish away their cancers, or that the mind can somehow treat cancer, if the patient only tries hard enough." One patient in Dr. Spiegel's research group dropped out of the group, stopped her chemotherapy and radiation, and decided only to do visualization practice to heal her cancer. She died within a year. This is profoundly upsetting to anyone, physician or relative. It neither proves nor disproves the possible value of visualization as an adjunct to conventional medical treatment. There is always the reality that many patients who complete their conventional treatment with chemotherapy and radiation also may die within the year.

Medical science can only speak of diseases, and not individual patients. This does not make either science or the patient right, or wrong. I have come to believe that there are no villains or heroes on the part of physicians and patients. There are people with highly technical skills and training, called physicians, and there are people with illnesses who consult the physicians, and then become patients. The degree to which their encounter becomes fruitful or successful will depend on several factors. One is internal, the patient's body. Another is external, the skills and knowledge of the physician, and thirdly the quality of the interaction between the two, the interpersonal chemistry. Support groups can frequently help individuals who are finding the interpersonal aspect of their medical or surgical treatment troublesome. Part of any physical healing includes both psychological and spiritual elements.

I received a letter from a member of the support group of which I have been a co-facilitator. She had requested a copy of her medical records from the oncologist's office. She wanted me to have a fuller understanding of her medical status, since she was living with a metastatic cancer. She sent them to me with a covering letter. In it she commented about her recent visit to the oncologists. She had seen a doctor who practices as a member of the group. She reported her experience as follows:

> Yesterday I had my big chemo, and felt awful, but better today. I saw Dr. K. I have heard a great deal about how good he is, and I believe he is top man there. Well, I went in with my list of questions and he refused absolutely to answer a single one of them. He kept saying, 'I pass on that one.' He had a strange way of looking you straight in the eye and never waivered. I like that up to a point, but it got to be too much. I waited almost an hour for him in a room with no heat, and I was frozen. I kept thinking he would return so I didn't say anything.
>
> I really have always hated to complain, but when I meet you, I do nothing else [she is referring to the support group and some individual meetings].
>
> I feel there is a big war going on between the holistic people and other doctors, particularly oncologists. I feel that the people with cancer are caught in the middle and left with fear and frustration. When I first had cancer (five years ago), I went to Dr. Siegel's lectures,

and many others. I bought about everything they had at ECaP and read and listened to tapes and got HOPE.

Then along came the oncologists, and they seemed to laugh at everything I then believed in. I even begged them to listen to some tapes and bought them and mailed them, but never even a thanks. I know they were angry. I have worked on Dr. Z. [her other oncologist in the office group] every time, but I think he doesn't go along with anything I say.

I feel badly about him, because I am just positive underneath there is such a warmth and a kind person. It shows in his eyes at times. I wish he could let a little of it out to his patients. I know his position is difficult. Cancer is an ugly thing and I don't think I can ever get to love mine. I just want to be healthy little bit longer. I have a lot of things I want to do. I have big ideas but run out of energy.

The patient completed a course of chemotherapy, and attended the support group faithfully every week, except when she and her husband were away for a vacation. Nine months after the letter quoted above, I asked her to write some comments about her support group experiences. She had attended one group in another city before coming to ours. Because her home was closer to ours than the first one, she sought out ours. She described her experiences:

I had had my lung fill up with fluid and had the tetracycline put in. I was feeling quite good about my health, but wanted to be in a group. This group had about twelve members. The same ones didn't always come and new ones would appear. I felt it was worth the long drive to get there. Charles [her husband] patiently went to shop or read in the car, as he never attended the group there. One of my daughters came once. She was so upset she had to go in the bathroom and cry.

Many of the people in that group were quite ill and four of them died. I felt awful about that as I have never really come to terms with my own, or anybody else's. I did feel very close to some of the members, and it was a place I could speak freely about my concerns. I liked P.[the facilitator] very much, but wished he could have said more.

My second support group [the author's] found me in a state of depression. The fluid I was told never would come back, did come back. I feel this support group is a wonderful thing.

Groups are a place where you can meet with people on another level than just social. We can talk about real concerns that our other friends wouldn't bother to listen to. We had one man in my first group who said he couldn't mention his cancer at home, and the group was the only place he could talk about it.

One man came only twice, but he told about being put on some kind of a new drug, and his doctor then told him he was cured. He had been very ill. We all rejoiced that he was well. A girl cried every time she came. She had a large tumor in her insides some place and they said they couldn't do anything for her. Finally she went to a doctor in Boston and he operated and she was fine. We rejoiced with her.

I can see an improvement in S.[another group member] every single week, and I am filled with joy for her and for B.[another group member]. It is wonderful to know such people.

When I ran groups before, I felt very close to the members [she had been a counselor herself before retirement]. I got more out of the groups than they did. People today are far too isolated. People need to realize they are a part of others and we all have problems. It is difficult to solve them alone, we need each other. A group is a place where you can cut away the pretense and get to know others.

Accompanying these comments was a covering letter, in which she closed by saying, "It has made a big difference in my life and in many ways I do bless the cancer for bringing it about." It may shock many who have had not had to deal personally with a serious illness to imagine that anyone could ever say anything positive about their illness, particularly cancer. This is not a rare comment. Since medical training defines disease as the arch-enemy, it would be difficult for many physicians to perceive disease in this manner, as having any positive value, meaning, or purpose.

This is not a criticism, only a comment. Another brief comment by a group member about the value of support groups stated that the group gave the participant ideas that were shared by others on how to deal with doctors, hospitals, fears, depression, and other topics. It was also mentioned that ideas derived from books, conferences, lectures were helpful. "Wouldn't hear about them if not in a group—chance to talk about and try out new ideas." I received a brief comment from another member who had attended our support group. He wrote the following:

> "Evaluation of group work—It is such a relief to find people who will listen to the vagaries of an illness, that is really listen, not interrupt, and give me the sense of entering into my experience. The slow leisurely pace of such disclosure is so supportive and somehow normalizes the pain. Pain shared with others becomes more tolerable. The feedback gives me courage to continue in a positive program. The weekly meetings become a real sustaining experience."

This man has been coping with a serious form of cancer, which included pain that required pain medication at times. His physicians could not give him an optimistic outlook for the future. He has also taken a large amount of responsibility for his own welfare, besides the regular medical treatments. He has made significant changes in his diet, exercised regularly, and continued actively to give help to many others, through friendship, counseling, and participation in several other groups. He is a young man in his seventies.

IV

*Twenty-First
Century Medicine*

17

Self-Responsibility and Partnership

The American Holistic Medical Association defines holistic medicine as "a philosophy of medical care that emphasizes personal responsibility and fosters a cooperative relationship among all those involved. It encompasses all safe modalities of diagnosis and treatment while emphasizing the whole person—physical, mental, emotional and spiritual. Life-style, environmental and nutritional factors are also considered." Conventional medicine does not specifically exclude any of these elements, nor should there be any conflict about these elements. The concept of personal responsibility by the patient is less emphasized, if at all, by the busy M. D. of today in conventional or cosmopolitan medical practice.

There is much discussion by physicians about "patient compliance" and the problems that occur when patients fail to follow the prescription as ordered by the doctor. But this is not what is usually meant by personal responsibility. Personal responsibility has more to do with the patient accepting responsibility for their own health and their own healing, with the active assistance of the doctor, to reach the goal of health. In strict legal terms, the physician is expected to render, through an "implied contract," proper diagnosis and treatment, to the best of her abilities, and in conformance with the prevailing practices of the medical community. Unfortunately too many citizens of late immediately assume that a "bad result" is the same as a failure to render adequate professional care. This is not the legal nor even moral requirement of any physician. If it were, he or she would then have to be God, since no physician or any other type of healer can guarantee results.

There are frequently stumbling-blocks for patients to take responsibility for themselves, and the state of their health. Responsibility, even in dictionary definitions, has the tone of being morally answerable, and therefore, blame and guilt can too easily be attached to the word. This has been the source of some criticism that has developed in response to some of Dr. Bernie Siegel's writings and lectures. There are milder negative reactions toward other professionals and writers who describe the contribution of emotional states and attitudes to the development of cancer and other major diseases.

A less commonly used meaning of "responsibility" in the American Heritage Dictionary is "capable of making moral or rational decisions on one's own," or "capable of being trusted or dependent upon; reliable." The words, reliance and self-reliance, might convey an additional aspect to what self-responsibility means. A responsible person is assumed to be someone who can make judgments about themselves or others. It does not follow automatically that any and all miscalculations deserve censure, criticism, or blame.

Another way of looking at this issue is to consider some opposite terms, such as victim or incompetent. "Blaming the victim" has been used as a phrase in critical attacks on Dr. Bernie Siegel and Dr. Carl Simonton, when they suggest that persons with cancer may have had personality factors that were involved in the onset of cancer. If a person is totally a victim, then it is true that they had no responsibility for the development of the disease. This also means that they are at the mercy of outside forces, relative to both cause and cure. There is no moral judgment or blame placed upon the environment or bacteria for being major causative factors in disease. It appears strange that any proposals that suggest internal, psychological factors as elements of cause immediately become colored with ethical qualities, including blame and guilt. It is true that some patients do express attitudes of guilt or blame, even without reading or hearing about self-contributing factors. This may have more to do with their inner tendencies to blame themselves for many other circumstances in life, besides their disease.

C. Norman Shealy, M. D. and Caroline M. Myss, M. A. in their provocative and intriguing book, *The Creation of Health* (Shealy & Myss, 1988) comment, "The position that it is the patient who is responsible for his/her healing process challenges the very core of the traditional medical paradigm, especially the doctor-patient relationship." Again we can see that the word, responsible has several different meanings. To be responsible can mean "to be in charge," despite any issue of outcome relating to blame or praise. Self-responsibility then suggests the wish and willingness to assert more power. There is a distinct difference in mental attitude between someone who believes there is nothing for them to do, nothing they can do, and that it is up to someone else, contrasted to someone who has the belief, and acts on it, that they can assert some degree of authority or power in what is happening.

I described briefly in the Chapter 2 a woman who fired her anesthesiologist when she was about to undergo surgery. This may not be the happiest example, but it at least points up the capacity for taking responsibility, i.e., empowering oneself, in a situation where most of us would not have imagined we could do so.

The increase in malpractice suits is at least partly attributed to the poor quality of relationship or communication between some patients and their doctors. Doctors for a variety of reasons, including increasing liability insurance costs, are working faster to see more patients, spending less time and having less good quality communication with their patients. As a result the patient then feels angry if there should be unsatisfactory, or even bad, results from treatment, and then are more prone to bring malpractice suits. This is self-perpetuating and painful for both physicians and patients. If a patient takes more responsibility, perhaps there might be less of a tendency to put all the outcome on the doctor's shoulders, and judge them in a less god-like way. It might also permit and encourage the physician not to have to act god-like. This also requires that the training of physicians also allows them to be comfortable not having to act in a manner that too easily is interpreted as "playing God."

Self-responsibility and self-empowerment by patients leads to another intimately connected issue of partnership. This is not a type or relationship for which doctors in conventional medicine have received any training or orientation. Many conventional physicians are open to being "trained" or reoriented by their patients, though it may require time and consideration. It can be done. In a weekly newspaper, *The Maine Times* (Austin, 1991), Phyllis Austin, a staff writer, presented a summary of her experiences following a nearly fatal accident. In an essay, "We must humanize medicine," she wrote (February 22, 1991):

> One of traditional medicine's aphorisms is that care of the patient requires caring for the patient. It's a "truth" I'm questioning because I've just been operated on and I was struck by my doctors' emotional disengagement. I needed comforting and compassion. Instead, they stood away from my bed as if we were strangers.
>
> I tried to imagine why they consciously avoided the human contact that I believe every patient has a "right" to expect from doctors. But anyway I looked at it, I couldn't accept that it was OK for my doctors to be emotionally neutral.
>
> Dr. Richard Rockefeller of Falmouth is an enlightening, empathetic physician with whom to talk about these matters; the touching/comforting issues are one of his primary interests. He teaches medical students and residents and encourages others to value the non-technical side of medicine, to approach patients with empathy, humor and hope—and to care about their uniqueness.
>
> To understand why health care has become so impersonal, Rockefeller cites the exponential growth of medical knowledge and technology over the past 75 years. "So tyrannized are physicians by this glut of information that comforting and caring have largely given way to memorization and procedural skills," he says. "Medical educators give lip service to traditional attributes of the healer—compassion, empathy, ethics and judgment among others— but the pressure to memorize leaves no time for explicitly teaching these, and there are few (doctor healers) left to serve as role models." "Neither do physicians receive time nor encouragement to deal with their own feelings in the face of the human suffering they confront daily," Rockefeller adds. "Many are numbed and come to ignore this realm, crucial though it is to effective practice and personal growth."
>
> For me, the doctor/patient relationship is more than an occasional subject. I see more of my doctors than I would like, given a near-death ski accident seven years ago. Since then, I have undergone repeated surgeries, thinking each one will be the last. But as my medical problems have continued, I've accepted that I'll likely have long-term dealings with doctors, in relationships that so far have been frustrating and imperfect.
>
> Much has been written about the benefits of shopping around for a doctor or surgeon to find the ideal one, especially in cases of serious disease and when the patient wants a physician to treat both body and soul. But in an accident or other medical emergency, such planning goes out the window.

In my case, I was taken to the nearest (rural) hospital and was treated by the doctor who happened to be on call. Too critical to talk, I was unconcerned about his bedside manner. The next surgery, within a few weeks of the first, also found me too ill to care. After two more operations, I knew the trauma and fears were adding up and I should pay attention to how humanistically my doctors were serving me.

But I hesitated. I didn't want to face the possibility of changing doctors in mid-treatment or going to a hospital far from home. I had no complaint about my doctors' procedural skills. They had given me excellent medical treatment, fixing what was wrong. The technical part of our 'contract' had been met.

Then came the fifth operation in January, when the need for my doctors to be compassionate and assuring couldn't be denied any longer. I wanted them to treat me with consideration for my injury history and the cumulative impact it has had on me. As well, I needed plain expressions of kindness—holding my hand and saying sympathetic words of support, telling me I'd be back on the top of mountains before long. But this was not to be.

I must interject that I had intended to assert myself in preparing for Round 5, to ask for what I needed point-blank. But last summer when I walked into my doctors' offices, I fell into the familiar pattern of the patient as the child and the doctor as the parent who knows all and knows best.

While I was sure my intestinal tract was malfunctioning, my doctors convinced me there was no reason to act hastily, despite my increasing pain and nausea. Since they had the medical degrees, their responses made me doubt my own 'unscientific' body knowledge. The fast-paced visits (in and out in 10 minutes) made me forget most or the informational questions I had about my condition or the surgical solution. And there was the not-so-small factor of fear of another operation and perhaps another after that, with each doctor giving me different prognoses.

By the first of the year, when waiting was no longer an option, I was firm with my surgeon on the subject of painkillers. I specifically asked for, and was told I would receive, the drug that worked best for me. But for the third operation in a row, I wasn't given what worked for me, a screw-up that told me my doctor wasn't listening to me. It was only after the intercession of friends, acting as patient advocates, that I received the right medication.

So what can any of us do to improve our experiences in a dehumanized medical system? There are a few steps Rockefeller suggests, noting, however, that the problems are so great and system-wide that "most solutions will be like small Band-Aids on a gushing wound." He advises patients to do everything possible "not to accept the child role that seems thrust upon them. Better health care results from collegial relationships, but not all doctors will take on patients as colleagues," he warns. "Establishing such a relationship sometimes requires patients even being a little obnoxious, even to the point of getting the physician mad with you."

My impulse is to work with the doctors I have, even if we have to have disagreements to come up with the kind of treatment partnership I want. I'm ready to be insistent and detailed, even if it gets down to telling them exactly what to do and say of a comforting nature. And even if our future meetings are just office visits, not surgical encounters, it would be an important shift in our relationship.

If I have to search for new doctors, I wonder if I should ask if they had had major surgery themselves, and know what it's like to lie in a hospital bed for weeks. Is that, ultimately, the easiest way to find doctors who, in living the life of a patient, treat the whole patient and not just the patient's body?

Illness and disease often create feelings of helplessness, dependency, and other qaualities we all have experienced as little children. The authority and responsibility that physicians are asked to assume easily stimulates strong parent-like qualities. Neither of these positions are intrinsically bad or harmful. Yet, the challenge is for both physicians and adult patients to be able to maintain a level of awareness and consciousness that does not produce poor parenting on the one hand or excessive childishness and helplessness on the other. A cooperative partnership can allow the best of a healing relationship to occur.

It has become too easy to collect horror stories from other citizens, similar to Phyllis Austin's experience. Simultaneously, I do not wish to support or propose any doctor-bashing, which can become a useless and destructive enterprise. The challenge for patients is to demand a share of responsibility for their treatment in a way that is not hostile, negative, or attacking. There is a clear difference between cold hostility and warm heart-felt anger in appropriate dosage. Once in a support group I was attending, a young woman with multiple sclerosis was describing her distress with her neurologist. She acknowledged that he was a highly competent, well-thought-of expert in his community, but she found his aloofness and distance so devastating that she was thinking seriously of leaving him. The group shared with her their thoughts about how she might challenge him in a loving way to be more human. This would require acting in a way that did not aggravate or scare him, and also avoided any erotic or sexualized behavior, or what he might construe as such. The young woman had never shared any of her distress with the neurologist himself. The group members raised the idea of very gently mentioning her distress without being hostile or challenging, but still honest. She also commented about his always sitting behind his large desk with her case file held up in front of him, and never touching her.

Two months later she reported to the group that she did speak with her neurologist. At the next visit after her sharing with him, she reported that he had placed his chair along the side of his desk with a more face-to-face conversation. As she was about to leave the office, he lightly put his hand on her shoulder, and she felt pleased that he was acting more human. She decided not to change doctors. Although the group often spoke of giving their doctors a hug, this young woman felt that she would have to wait awhile, so as not to scare her doctor back behind his desk. Some people, whether doctor or patient, can be very touchy about being touched or hugged, and some degree of sensitivity is needed in changing social behavior.

On another occasion a woman who attended a support group that I was co-facilitating told about her experience with an oncologist who had been treating her for the past year. She reported that he had an outstanding reputation as a very competent and well-trained specialist in the region. She reported, however that every time she left his office she felt worse, because he conveyed such a depressing and discouraging manner and didn't take any time to answer her questions. She drove two hours to reach his office, and often waited at least an hour before she saw him. Initially she spoke as if she believed she didn't have any options at all. No direct advice or recommendations were given to her by the group or the group facilitators.

She was asked if she had thought at all of seeing if there were an oncologist closer to home who also might be satisfactory. She returned the next week with a wonderful smile, and reported that she "just happened to" hear that a new oncologist was now available within a half-hour of her home. She had made an appointment to see if she could work with him. To her delight she found him to be everything she had wanted in a competent physician, with a more pleasant manner and apparently competent in his professional knowledge. She made a peaceful and friendly disengagement with her previous doctor. Over the following year she has maintained her health despite her disease, with no symptoms of illness.

There is no question that even the most traditional of conventional physicians would be delighted to see all of their patients take responsibility for their health, in contrast to disease or illness. This is an area where physicians have difficulty finding ways to mobilize self-responsibility. The major elements for holislic health, or health in general, relate to nutrition, exercise, stress reduction and life-style. As previously mentioned the leading causes of death relate to life-style. Overeating, overdrinking, smoking, and over-the-speed-limit driving cause disease and death on a massive scale. The cartoon character, Pogo, has frequently been quoted as saying, "We have met the enemy and they are us."

The field of behavioral medicine carried out mostly by Ph. D. psychologists, has developed strategies to help people find healthier ways to live. Group programs to help people lose weight, stop smoking, give up alcohol and drug abuse are increasingly available. The major problem for many individuals is motivation, choosing to participate. The maintenance of good health is still far from a central part of most people's consciousness in the United States and many other industrialized nations. Affluence does not proportionally increase health or contribute to less disease. In fact, the evidence keeps accumulating that the opposite is true.

Prevention is a term that is easily bandied about, but there is very little energy or money spent in the health field for it. Almost no "health" insurance is available for maintaining health. The correct term should be "illness" or "disease" insurance, but that does not sound as pleasant. There are very few insurance programs that financially reward people for staying healthy. Some corporations have developed rewards for employees if they don't take sick days, or do not use their medical insurance. One company gave a financial bonus to employees who walked up sixteen flights of stairs to the office, instead of using the elevator. There is an insurance company in Holland that gives a reduced rate for medical insurance to policyholders who practice meditation regularly. These are small items compared to the bulk of the medical insurance field, which is geared only to disease treatment reimbursements.

This brings the challenge back to the individual and his or her choices. It does not require a psychic to know that we are more than the parts and pieces that surgeons can remove. This is a key point in holistic medicine and health. We are not only bodies, but minds, hearts, and souls. Both physicians and patients must find an approach that allows both to share their journeys as they meet each other. The meeting would respect each of these elements.

18
Conclusion

A conclusion is both an ending and a decision. The legal definition describes a conclusion as the close of a plea or deed. In its simplest terms, it is the last chapter of a book, a summing up. It is also a statement of what the implications are, an opinion. The entire book has been a series of opinions more than absolute facts, with a scattering of scientific facts here and there. The purpose and goal have been to inform the reader there are many possibilities that exist for the maintenance of health, and for the healing of ailments.

A contribution from the Eastern traditions of philosophy and medicine is yin and yang, a set of opposites that are not antagonistic or in conflict, but simply complementary to each other. Each is the inside out of the other. This concept is a useful instrument for thinking about holistic medicine and conventional, scientific medicine. They need not be at odds with each other, and they can each bring distinctive viewpoints and methods to the other. British medicine has usually called holistic methods *complementary medicine*.

We in the modern, "Western" traditions of medicine have become trained in rational, measurable ways of thinking. It is not easy to allow room simultaneously for another more intuitive, non-rational approach to health and healing. The older traditions of healing in the East, i.e., China, Japan, and India, have been partially replaced by the modern scientific viewpoint. These countries also can comfortably co-exist with their traditional systems. They never disappeared completely. For Americans and Europeans, it is more difficult to be comfortable with viewpoints that had once been part of the culture, but have now been replaced by more scientifically oriented approaches in the past one or two hundred years. The roots of these scientific principles have been growing for two thousand years of history since Hippocrates. The empirical and folk methods have been violently suppressed. The first holocaust may well have been the execution of several million women who were accused of being witches because they practiced herbal medicine. Every small village throughout Europe had at least one or two women who knew the use of herbs. They were ready targets during the infamous witch hunts of the fourteenth and fifteenth centuries.

I am not proposing abandonment of the scientifically grounded medicine of the twentieth century. Still, I do suggest there can be some usefulness in considering the various methods that this book describes. This does require some risk-taking that each person must consider for themselves. There are, at least for now, few statistics that can easily support nonconventional approaches. There is greater safety when they are a supplement to conventional medical care, or when used only for health maintenance or prevention. If used without active involvement of conventional medicine, there are greater risks.

I recently received a letter from the grieving sister of a woman I had met six years ago. Her sister informed me that my friend, R., had died of cancer six months earlier. I had written R. a few months before to ask how she was, not knowing she had already died. My letter was found unopened among her possessions. I had never met the sister, but my letter moved her to write to me. She informed me how upset she had been that her sister had refused conventional medical care for her cancer, except initially. Instead she had chosen to follow a special nutritional approach.

When I first met R., she told me that the cancer was in an advanced stage, with metastasis from breast cancer to sixteen lymph nodes. Six months earlier she received the diagnosis. She underwent a lumpectomy. She then sought out the advice of two of the most well-known oncologists on the East Coast. Neither gave her much hope but did recommend what was currently available, radiation and chemotherapy. After studying the proposals as carefully as she could, as a well-educated layperson, she decided not to proceed further with the recommendations. She would follow her own path.

At the time I first met her, she showed me her hands, which revealed distinctive discolorations. I had read about this but had never actually seen it before this time. There were green and yellow streaks present that can occur in advanced cancers. Her mood was cheerful and optimistic when we first met, and on all later occasions. She had been on a special dietary program for about six months. She also had involved herself in several other activities that were supportive to her both physically and emotionally.

As a physician it was the first time I had ever met someone with a serious and obvious life-threatening condition, who was not choosing to follow a reasonable and rational medical treatment. I need to add there were no signs or comments that suggested she was suffering from any serious psychiatric disorder, nor any other hints to suggest questioning her competency to make choices.

I acknowledge that I had grave reservations about her decision. I did not know then what the statistics would be for her from a conventional standpoint. In thinking about her and her sister's understandable distress over the choices she made, I recall now the research by Dr. David Spiegel I mentioned in the chapter on support groups. In his study of eighty-six women with metastatic breast cancer, most of them had died within eighteen to forty-one months from time of diagnosis. All had undergone complete standard medical and surgical treatment. Some had received additional group therapy. What is vivid in this study is the relatively short survival time of less than four years, except for three women who were alive ten years later. I have no way of determining if R. might have lived longer if she had agreed to additional medical care after lumpectomy.

She did live almost five and a half years with only lumpectomy. When I met her in three successive years, she looked increasingly healthy and energetic. She carried on an active and normal life until her last six to twelve months. I appreciate that I do not have the complete medical findings to make a valid clinical judgment, except for the facts R. presented, and the obvious severity of her condition from the beginning. I do not suggest that any physician could support what she did. It does raise many unanswerable questions. I spoke with her sister by telephone, after receiving the letter.

She shared with me that R. had avoided any kind of medical care, including pain-killers and any medical treatment that might have given her some pain relief and perhaps some questionable extension of life. I heard the distress beyond the grief of losing a sister. She felt that R. had been excessively caught up in the belief system of this nutritional approach that saw no value whatsoever in conventional medical care. R.'s sister had strong reasons to question the honesty and integrity of the advisors who had counseled her sister, because they were so zealous and absolute in their advice to R., including no suggestion, when R. was obviously beginning to deteriorate rapidly, that any medical care be obtained. I could not argue against a need for more flexibility and more humility by R.'s nutritional advisors. It is extremely difficult for any family member to give a patient support, if a person chooses an unconventional type of treatment that the family cannot understand or appreciate. In R.'s circumstances, she was a strong-willed person who had an intense faith in what she was doing, even when she could no longer see any positive results.

The harsh question remains "what is reality?" or "whose reality?" Perhaps R. lived longer through the path she took, and had a more satisfying quality of life, despite the actual physical pain she endured in her last six to twelve months of life. On the other hand, her sister and many others would see her choice as foolish, unrealistic, and leading to her death more certainly than if she had been less adventuresome, and had followed doctors' orders. There are no scientific experiments or studies that can be acceptable when only one person is the subject of the study. In scientific circles, this is called "an n of 1."

The "n" stands for the numbers in the experiment. A scientific study requires several subjects to be compared or contrasted to another group, treated and untreated. I once heard a research scientist tell me about an experiment he did on a single rat. He told me he had succeeded in creating a situation in which a rat acted in a way that was the equivalent of suicide. I do not recall the specifics of the experiment, but he reported that the rat did behave in a way that caused its own death. He commented to me that he doubted he could report the experiment since "one suicidal rat is not a scientific study." As far as I know, he never reported his single, or n=1, experiment to any scientific journals. This is the perpetual problem of anecdotal reports.

I mention R. not because she appears to have been a clear success nor a failure. I only knew her briefly over a four-year period. Despite the brevity of our contacts, she had an unusual amount of unself conscious caring and love toward the people she met. Despite her serious illness, she always conveyed a striking sparkle in her personality. Her sister informed me that she had been active and enjoying life until the last year, when she began to slip downhill. Her death and the loss to her family saddens me. I reserve judgment in declaring if she was foolish for being so set against conventional treatment, or if she was adventuresome and sensible in getting what she wanted for herself—to a degree—at a price. I know she wanted to achieve a long-lasting remission, in the face of overwhelming odds. She obtained only a partial one.

In the now classic Japanese movie, *Rashomon*, three versions of a traumatic event, a crime, are presented through the eyes of the victim, the perpetrator, and a witness. There are three versions of reality.

Holistic medicine and conventional medicine are two forms of reality, as are poetry and prose. Perhaps in the coming decades there can be a blending of both that will contribute to health for more people, and additional ways for healing of illness and disease. The severe financial stresses that are occurring in the United States for increasing numbers of citizens seeking health and medical care are approaching a breaking-point. The challenge for holistic medicine is to contribute to some solutions for easing the burdens on the health-care system. Beyond this specific problem, there is a need to find additional health-care methods to aid the less industrialized countries of the world who cannot readily supply their citizens with modern, conventional medical care. Less technological ways of healing that are effective will make a contribution.

A final point is the large cultural diversity now within the United States and many European countries. Many cities in the United States have population groups that are highly diverse in their cultural backgrounds. This diversity includes medical care systems and belief systems different from conventional modern, technological medical care. For many who have come from Southeast Asia, China, various Central American countries, and many other diverse cultures, there needs to be an appreciation of these belief systems. A holistic orientation can be sensitive to the non-technological needs valued in these cultures by those who have grown up in them.

There is an increasing need for blending East and West, North and South.

Bibliography

Achterberg, Jeanne. *Imagery in Healing: Shamanism and Modern Medicine.* Boston: New Science Library, 1985.

Altenberg, Henry. "My Explorations in Macrobiotics." *Doctors Look at Macrobiotics.* Ed. Edward Esko. Tokyo & New York: Japan Publications, Inc., 1988.

Anderson, Greg. *The Cancer Conqueror: An Incredible Journey to Wellness.* Kansas City, MO: Andrews and McMeel, 1990.

Ardell, Donald B. *High Level Wellness.* Emmaus, PA: Rodale Press, 1977.

Assagioli, Roberto. *Psychosynthesis.* New York: Viking, 1965.

Baginski, Bodo, and Shalila Sharamon. *Reiki: Universal Life Energy.* Mendocino, California: LifeRhythm, 1988.

Benson, Herbert, and Miriam Z. Klipper. *The Relaxation Response.* New York: Avon Books, 1976.

———, and William Proctor. *Beyond the Relaxation Response.* New York: Berkley, 1985.

"BOIRON's Hallmark of quality: Its 60-year Quest for Proof." *Prescriber.* V: 4. Norwood, PA: BOIRON Educational Institute, 1991.

Borysenko, Joan. *Minding the Body, Mending the Mind.* Reading, MA: Addison-Wesley Publishing Co., 1987.

Brown, Malcolm. *The Healing Touch: An Introduction to Organismic Psychotherapy.* Mendocino, California: LifeRhythm, 1990.

Boucher, Joseph. "Naturopathic Medicine: a Separate and Distinct Healing Profession." *Wholisic Dimensions in Healing.* Ed. Leslie J. Kaslof. New York: Doubleday, 1978.

Capra, Fritjof. *The Tao of Physics.* New York: Bantam Books, 1975.

———. *The Turning Point.* New York: Bantam Books, 1983.

Chopra, Deepak. *Perfect Health: The Complete Mind/Body Guide.* New York: Harmony Books, 1990.

Colbin, Annemarie. *Food and Healing.* New York: Ballantine, 1986.

———. *The Book of Whole Meals.* New York: Ballantine, 1983.

A Course in Miracles. Tiburon, CA: Foundation for Inner Peace, 1975.

Cousins, Norman. *The Anatomy of an Illness.* New York: W.W. Norton, 1979.

Crampton, Martha. "Psychological Energy Transformations: Developing Positive Polarization." *Transpersonal Psychology* 6.1 (1974)

Cummings, Stephen, and Dana Ullman. *Everybody's Guide to Homeopathic Medicine*. Los Angeles: Jeremey P. Tarcher, Inc., 1984.

Diamond, John. *Behavioral Kinesiology*. New York: Harper and Row, 1979.

Eisenberg, David, with Thomas Lee Wright. *Encounters with Qi: Exploring Chinese Medicine*. New York: W.W. Norton, 1985.

Epstein, Gerald. *Healing Visualizations: Creating Health Through Imagery*. New York: Bantam Books, 1989.

Engel, George L. "The need for a new medical model: A challenge for biomedicine." *Science* 196: 129, 1977.

——. "The Clinical Application of the Biopsychosocial Model." *American Journal of Psychiatry*. 127: 535 (1980).

Farquhar, John W. *The American Way of Life Need Not Be Hazardous to Your Health*. New York: W.W. Norton, 1978.

Fiore, Neil. "Fighting Cancer-One Patient's Perspective." *The New England Journal of Medicine*. 300: 284–289 (1979).

——. *The Road Back to Health: Coping with the Emotional Aspects of Cancer*. Berkeley, California: Celestial Arts, 1990.

Flach, Frederic. *Rickie*. New York: Fawcett Columbine, 1990.

Frawley, David. *Ayurvedic Healing*. Salt Lake City, Utah: Passage Press, 1989.

——, and Vasant Lad. *The Yoga of Herbs*. Santa Fé, New Mexico: Lotus Press, 1985.

Furth, Gregg. *Secret World of Drawings: Healing through Art*. Boston: Sigo Press, 1988.

Gerber, Richard. *Vibrational Medicine*. Santa Fé, New Mexico: Bear and Company, 1988.

Gordon, James. *Holistic Medicine*. New York: Chelsea House Publishers, 1988.

Haberly, Helen. *Hawayo Takata's Story*. Garrett Park, Maryland: Archedigm, 1990.

Hammer, Leon. *Dragon Rises, Red Bird Flies*. New York: Station Hill Press, 1990.

Hay, Louise L. *You Can Heal Life*. Santa Monica, California: Hay House, 1984.

Heimlich, Jane. *What Your Doctor Won't Tell You*. New York: Harper Collins, 1990.

Heyn, Birgit. *Ayurveda: The Indian Art of Natural Medicine and Life Extension*. Rochester, Vermont: Healing Arts Press, 1983.

Inglis. Brian. *The Case for Unorthodox Medicine*. New York: Berkeley, 1969.

Jampolsky, Gerald G. *Love is Letting Go of Fear*. Berkeley, California: Celestial Arts, 1979.

——. *Out of Darkness, Into the Light*. New York: Bantam Books, 1989.

Kabat-Zinn, Jon. *Full Catastrophe Living: Using the Wisdom of Your Body and Mind to Face Stress, Pain and Illness*. New York: Delacorte Press, l990.

Kaptchuk, Ted J. *The Web That Has No Weaver*. New York: Congdon and Weed, 1983.

Krieger, Dolores. *The Therapeutic Touch: How to Use Your Hands to Help and Heal*. Englewood Cliffs, NJ: Prentice Hall, 1979.

Kubler-Ross, Elizabeth. *On Death and Dying*. New York: MacMillan, 1969.

Kushi, Michio. *Crime and Diet: The Macrobiotic Approach*. Tokyo & New York: Japan Publications, Inc., 1987.

——, and Phillip Jannetta. *Macrobiotics and Oriental Medicine*. Tokyo & New York: Japan Publications, Inc., 1991.

——, with Olivia Oredson. *Macrobiotic Palm Healing: Energy at Your Finger-tips*. Tokyo & New York: Japan Publications, Inc., 1988.

Lad, Vasant. *Ayurveda: The Science of Self-Healing*. Santa Fé. NM: Lotus Press, 1984.

Lappe Frances Moore. *Diet for a Small Planet*. New York: Ballantine, 1971.

Leonard, Jim and Phil Laut. *Rebirthing: The Science of Enjoying All of Your Life*. Hollywood, CA: Trinity Publications, 1983.

LeShan, Lawrence. *Cancer as a Turning Point*. New York: E.P. Dutton, 1990.

——. *How to Meditate*. New York: Bantam Books, 1974.

Lock, Margaret. *East Asian Medicine in Urban Japan*. Berkeley, CA: University of California Press, 1980.

Lowen, Alexander. *Bioenergetics*. New York: Penguin Books, 1976.

——. "Some Notes About Cancer." *Bioenergetic Analysis*. 3: 1 (1987)

Lucas, Richard. *Nature's Medicines*. No. Hollywood, CA: Wilshire Book Co., 1974.

Matthews-Simonton, Stephanie. *The Healing Family*. New York: Bantam Books, 1984.

McDougall, John A. *McDougall's Medicine, a Challenging Second Opinion*. Piscataway, NJ: New Century Publications, Inc., 1985.

——. *The McDougall Plan*. Piscataway, NJ: New Century Publications, Inc., 1983.

Norris, Patricia and Garrett Porter. *Why Me?: Harnessing the Healing Power of the Human Spirit*. Walpole, NH: Stillpoint Publishing, 1985.

Northrop, F.S.C. *The Meeting of East and West*. New York: The MacMillan Co., 1946.

Orr, Leonard and Sondra Ray. *Rebirthing In the New Age*. Berkeley, California: Celestial Arts, 1977.

Oyle, Irving. *The Healing Mind: You Can Cure Yourself Without Drugs*. Millbrae, California: Celestial Arts, 1975.

——. *Time, Space and the Mind*. Millbrae, California: Celestial Arts, 1976.

Pelletier, Kenneth. *Holistic Medicine: From Stress to Optimum Health*. New York: Delacorte and Delta, 1979.

Pfeiffer, Carl C. *Mental and Elemental Nutrients*. New Canaan, CT: Keats Publishing, Inc., 1975.

Ram Das. *Be Here Now*. New York: Crown Publishing, 1971.

——. *The Only Dance There Is*. New York: Anchor Press, 1974.

Ray, Sondra. *Celebration of Breath*. Berkeley, California: Celestial Arts, 1983.

Reich, Wilhelm. *The Cancer Biopathy*. New York: Farrar, Straus and Giroux, 1973.

Robbins, John. *Diet for a New America*. Walpole, NH: Stillpoint Publishing, 1987.

Samuels, Mike and Nancy Samuels. *Seeing with the Mind's Eye*. New York: Random House, 1975.

—— and Harold Bennett. *The Well Body Book*. New York: Random House, 1973.

Sandler, Stephen. *Osteopathy, the Illustrated Guide*. New York: Harmony Books, 1989.

Sattilaro, Anthony. *Recalled By Life*. Boston: The Houghton Mifflin Co., 1982.

Shealy, C. Norman and Caroline M. Myss. *The Creation of Health*. Walpole, NH: Stillpoint Publishing, 1988.

Siegel, Bernard. *Love. Medicine and Miracles*. New York: Harper and Row, 1986.

——. *Peace, Love and Healing*. New York: Harper and Row, 1989.

Simonton Carl and Stephanie Matthews-Simonton. *Getting Well Again*. New York: Bantam Books, 1980.

Spiegel, David, et al. "Effect of Psychosocial Treatment on Survival of Patients with Metastatic Breast Cancer." *Lancet* 14 Oct. 1989: 888–891.

——. "A Psychosocial Intervention and Survival Time of Patients with Metastatic Breast Cancer." *Advances The Journal of Mind-Body Health* 7: 3 (Summer 1991)

"The Surgeon General's Report on Nutrition and Health: The Summary and Recommendations." New York: Warner Books, 1989.

Svoboda, Robert E. *Prakruti: Your Ayurvedic Constitution*. Albuquerque, NM: Geocom, 1989.

——. *The Hidden Secret of Ayurveda*. Pune, India: n.p., 1980.

Tara, William. *Macrobiotics and Human Behavior*. Tokyo & New York: Japan Publications, Inc., 1985.

Tisserand, Robert. *The Art of Aromatherapy*. Rochester, Vermont: Healing Arts Press, 1977.

Tribe, Bill. "Naturopathic Medicine." *The Holistic Health Handbook*. Berkeley, California: And/or Press, 1978.

Tsumura, Akira. *Kampo: How the Japanese Updated Traditional Herbal Medicine*. Tokyo & New York: Japan Publications, Inc., 1991.

Veith, Ilza. *Nei Ching: The Yellow Emperor's Classic of Internal Medicine*. Berkeley, CA: University of California Press, 1972.

Walford, Roy L. *Maximum Life Span*. New York: W.W. Norton, 1983.

——. *The 120 Year Diet: How to Double Your Vital Years*. New York: Simon and Schuster, 1986.

Watts, Alan W. *Psychotherapy East and West*. New York: Ballantine Books, 1961.

Weeks, Nora. *The Medical Discoveries of Edward Bach, Physician*. New Canaan, CT: Keats Publishing Co., 1979.

Weil, Andrew. *Health and Healing*. Boston: Houghton Mifflin, 1986.

——. *Natural Health. Natural Medicine*. Boston: Houghton Mifflin, 1990.

Wild, Richard. "Chiropractic." *Hands-On Healing*. Ed. John Feltman. Emmaus, Pennsylvania: Rodale Press, 1989.

Wilhelm, Richard. *The I Ching*. Princeton, NJ: Princeton University Press, 1967.

Wisneski, Leonard A. "The Pineal Gland: Our Window to the Biosphere." Annual Scientific Conference AHMA Seattle, WA,

Yamamoto, Shizuko. *Barefoot Shiatsu*. Tokyo & New York: Japan Publications, Inc., 1979.

Reading Recommendations

Altenberg, Henry. "My Explorations in Macrobiotics." *Doctors Look at Macrobiotics*. Ed. Edward Esko. Tokyo & New York: Japan Publications, Inc., 1988. (Also, reprinted in *Macrobiotics Today*. July/August 1990 vol. 30, No. 4)

Anderson, Greg. *The Cancer Conqueror: An Incredible Journey to Wellness*. Kansas City, MO: Andrews and McMeel, 1990.

Chopra, Deepak. *Quantum Healing: Exploring the Frontiers of Mind/Body Medicine*. New York: Bantam Books 1989.

Colbin, Annemarie. *Food and Healing*. New York: Ballantine, 1986.

A Course in Miracles. Tiburon. CA: Foundation for Inner Peace, 1975.

Dufty, William. *Sugar Blues*. New York: Warner Books, 1976.

Hay, Louise L. *You Can Heal Your Life*. Santa Monica, California: Hay House, 1984.

Jampolsky, Gerald G. *Love is Letting Go of Fear*. Berkeley, California: Celestial Arts, 1979.

Kabat-Zinn, Jon. *Full Catastrophe Living: Using the Wisdom of Your Body and Mind to Face Stress Pain and Illnes*s. New York: Delacorte Press, 1990.

McDougall, John. *The McDougall Plan*. Piscataway, NJ: New Century Publications, Inc., 1983.

Robbins, John. *Diet For a New America*. Walpole, NH: Stillpoint Publishing, 1987.

Siegel, Bernard. *Love, Medicine and Miracles*. New York: Harper and Row, 1986.

Weil, Andrew. *Natural Health, Natural Medicine*. Boston: Houghton Mifflin, 1990.

A Few Resources

To obtain further information, literature, or names and addresses of practitioners, you may wish to contact some of the following:

Acupuncture and Chinese Medicine
American College of Traditional Chinese
  Medicine
455 Arkansas Street
San Francisco, CA 94107

New England School of Acupuncture
30 Common Street
Watertown, MA 02172

The School of T'ai Chi Ch'uan, Inc.
47 West 13th ST.
New York, NY 10011

Ayurveda
American Association of Ayurvedic
  Medicine
P.O. Box 541
Lancaster, MA
01523

The Ayurveda
Institute
1131 Menaul,
N.E. Suite A
Albuquerque, NM 87112

Yoga Journal
California Yoga Journal Association
2054 University Avenue
Berkeley, CA 94704

Bioenergetic Analysis
Institute for
Bioenergetic
Analysis
144 East 36 Street
New York, NY 10016

Institute for Bioenergetics and Gestalt
1307 University Avenue
Berkeley, CA 94702

Chiropractic
American Chiropractic Association
1701 Clarendon Blvd.
Arlington, VA 22209

International College of Applied
  Kinesiology
P.O. Box 25276
Shawnee Mission, KS 66225

Herbalism

American Herb Association
P.O. Box 353
Rescue, CA 95672

American Aromatherapy Association
P.O. Box 1222
Fair Oaks, CA 95628

Holistic Medicine

American Holistic Medical Association
4101 Lake Boone Trail, Suite 201
Raleigh, NC 27607

Homeopathy

Dr. Edward Bach Healing Society
P.O. Box 320
Woodmere, NY 11598

Flower Essence Society
P.O. Box 459
Nevada City, CA 95959

Homeopathic Educational Services
2124 Kittridge Street
Berkeley, CA 94704

National Center for Homeopathy
1500 Massachusetts Avenue N.W., Suite 42
Washington, D.C. 20005

Macrobiotics

Kushi Institute of the Bershires
Box 7
Becket, MA 01223

Vega Study Center
1511 Robinson Street
Oroville, CA 95965

Massage

American Massage Therapy
  Association
National Information Office
1130 West North Shore Avenue
Chicago, IL 60626

Medicine

American Medical Association
515 N. State Street
Chicago, IL 60610

Naturopathy

American Association of Naturopathic
  Physicians
P.O. Box 20386
Seattle, WA 98102

John Bastyr College of Naturopathic
  Medicine
144 N.E. 54 Street
Seattle, WA 98105

National College of Naturopathic Medicine
11231 S.E. Market Street
Portland, OR 97216

Nutrition

North American Vegetarian Society
P.O. Box 72
Dodgerville, NY 13329

Osteopathy

American Osteopathy Association
142 East Ontario
Chicago, IL 60611

Polarity Therapy

American Polarity Therapy Association
P.O. Box 44-154
West Somerville, MA 02144

Reiki

Radiance Association
P.O. Box 40570-0570
St. Petersburg, FL 33743

Reiki Alliance
P.O. Box 41
Cataldo, ID 83810

Support Groups

American Cancer Society
777 Third Avenue
New York, NY 10017

> CanSurmount
> I Can Cope } programs available
> through ACS
> Reach to Recovery

Candlelighters
1901 Pennsylvania Avenue NW
Washington, DC 20003

Center for Attitudinal Healing
19 Main Street
Tiburon, CA 94920 (415–435–5022)

ECaP
1302 Chapel Street
New Haven, CT 06511
(203–865–8392)

H.O.P.E.
52 High Street
South Paris, ME 04281

Make Today Count
P.O. Box 303
Burlington, Iowa 52601

Therapeutic Touch

Nurse Healers-Professional Association,
  Inc.
175 Fifth Ave., Suite 3399
New York, NY 10010

Index